FREEDOM

FROM STRONGHOLDS

WORKBOOK

Printed in the United States of America
Remnant Publishing

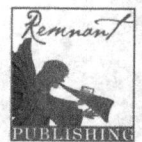

WeighDown Ministries ®
Brentwood, Tennessee 37024
1-800-844-5208
www.weighdown.com

ISBN # 978-1-892729-40-8

NOW THE LORD IS THE SPIRIT,
AND WHERE THE SPIRIT OF
THE LORD IS,
THERE IS FREEDOM.
II CORINTHIANS 3:17

THIS BOOK BELONGS TO:

_____

BEFORE YOU BEGIN...

You may have joined this program because of strongholds or addictions that have had an impact upon your body as well as your spirit. If this is the case, we recommend that you consult your physician or counselor for an examination and to address any individual concerns before you begin. Also, if you have any preexisting health conditions, please continue to remain under your physician's care. Reducing the intake of excessive amounts of alcohol, medication, food, etc., will be a positive change, but the body that has become accustomed to excess may experience some unfamiliar feelings during the transition. God has made our bodies to be sensitive to what and how much of anything we need, but this internal system must be resurrected! Be patient and trust God to ultimately satisfy you far better than anything the world can offer.

This seminar was developed to address the heart's addiction and dependence upon the things of the world as a comfort and a delight. Jesus stated the most important commandment was to love the Lord our God with all our heart, soul, mind, and strength (Mark 12:28-29), not give our heart and soul and mind to substances or things on this Earth. Ephesians 5:18 warned the early Christians not to get drunk on wine but to "be filled with the Spirit." These Christians did not have access to antidepressants as we know them today, but the principle is the same. God's people have adopted an alarming stance on the liberal use of pharmaceuticals and recreational drugs for the pain of an undirected heart. Instead of heeding the warning to stop loving something on this Earth, we have embraced medications and other substances to numb the symptoms of sin—to a fault.

It is all too inviting to assume that our emotions or physical feelings are caused by something beyond our control or some chemical malfunction. While of course this is the case in some situations, a true chemical imbalance is the exception rather than the rule. Excessive use of medication/substances, food, or alcohol to counteract the imbalance in our obedience to God provides only temporary, artificial relief. However, we have witnessed thousands of people reexamine their hearts to discover that true deliverance is found when they stop investing their lives in the idols of this Earth and begin to reinvest their lives in loving God Almighty, looking to Him as primary source of comfort and direction.

Again, if you currently have any condition that causes you concern or has an impact on your body and/or spirit, we recommend that you consult your physician or counselor for an examination and to address any individual concerns before you begin. Also, if you have any preexisting health conditions, please continue to remain under your physician's care to best treat your personal situation.

TABLE OF CONTENTS

INTRODUCTION 6

1. SET FREE FROM PAIN 19

2. GOD'S BOUNDARIES 33

3. CLEAR-MINDED AND SELF-CONTROLLED 51

4. FREEDOM OF THE MIND 67

5. PURITY OF FOCUS 79

6. A JOYFUL SPIRIT 93

7. A LIFE OF PEACE 105

8. FREE TO LOVE GOD 121

APPENDIX 134

INTRODUCTION
FREEDOM BASICS

The Spirit of the Sovereign Lord is on me, because the Lord has anointed me to preach good news to the poor. He has sent me to bind up the broken-hearted, to proclaim freedom for the captives and release from darkness for the prisoners... Isaiah 61:1

Therefore do not let anyone judge you by what you eat or drink, or with regard to a religious festival, a New Moon celebration or a Sabbath day. These are a shadow of the things that were to come; the reality, however, is found in Christ. Do not let anyone who delights in false humility and the worship of angels disqualify you for the prize. Such a person goes into great detail about what he has seen, and his unspiritual mind puffs him up with idle notions. He has lost connection with the Head, from whom the whole body, supported and held together by its ligaments and sinews, grows as God causes it to grow. Since you died with Christ to the basic principles of this world, why, as though you still belonged to it, do you submit to its rules: "Do not handle! Do not taste! Do not touch!"? These are all destined to perish with use, because they are based on human commands and teachings. Such regulations indeed have an appearance of wisdom, with their self-imposed worship, their false humility and their harsh treatment of the body, but they lack any value in restraining sensual indulgence. Colossians 2:16-23

You are about to embark on a unique journey of freedom. It is a journey away from the magnetic pull of any stronghold that has a hold on your heart and mind. At the same time, it is a journey toward replacing this stronghold with a new stronghold—God Almighty—who has all resources for anything you need and is the source of all feelings that can fill up your heart. You are not a failure. Years of misguided counseling and gimmicks have only increased your attraction and allegiance toward your strongholds. Again, you are not a failure! You have just been trying to free yourself with man's suggestions, and they have only driven you deeper into yourself and gratifying your own desires.

It does not matter what it is that brought you here. God does not look at the outside. God looks at the heart. We know that your heart is searching to please the Lord God Almighty, the Ruler of the Heavens and the Earth, and that is all that matters to us! You need to understand that you CAN do this, and the reason that the lies that discourage you by saying things like "you are not going to make it" or "you are no good" are so loud and the war is so intense is because **you** are so incredibly valuable. You do not even realize the value of the price tag on your head. God has brought you to this Series today for a reason. The Spirit of God will be over you and in you, and I pray it is so impactful that you will never be the same after today.

You are about to join a mighty exodus of people who are choosing to walk away from slavery to their old habits. This miserable state of slavery is not unlike the bondage the children of God felt when they were

---

THE LORD OUR GOD CAN DELIVER YOU FROM ANY ADDICTION THAT HAS A HOLD ON YOU.

---

enslaved centuries ago to the Egyptian pharaohs. The Old Testament story of the Exodus tells how God's children, once subjugated to Pharaoh, were forced into slave labor to build Egyptian structures. Those towering icons are representations of the strength and the soul that they invested in Egypt. At one time, His children were free men in a foreign land. When God saw that they had become slaves to making bricks for Egypt and heard their cries, He fought a mighty battle for the deliverance of the Israelites.

He is fighting now for the deliverance of your heart so that you will no longer be overpowered by those things that seem to control you and drain you of your health, your energy, your time, your relationships, your joy—even your very life. The Lord our God can deliver you from any addiction that has a hold on you. You are not undisciplined—you have just not tried this approach to breaking free.

So we have all started off behind bars or in Egypt—enslaved with an imprisoned heart—because we have given our devotion to something on this Earth. Since we are slaves to what we love, it will take an even stronger love to remove us. God let the Israelites know that He would not sit by and let Egypt enslave them. He exposed Egypt for what it was...worthless. He showed His passionate, jealous love and power in an incredible display of devastating plagues. The Israelites made the right choice and followed Him out of Egypt, into the desert, and finally into the Promised Land. In this Series, we hope that the prison scenes will make you aware of the spiritual bars that surround you—exposing your enslavement for what it is.

Our Egypt may seem different, but being locked into an affair or pornography, battling an addiction to alcohol, food, nicotine, or drugs, or being controlled by financial debt or anger or online gaming is equally enslaving. We have given our strength and our soul to something on this Earth, and it has become our master. Even if it seems as "small" as anger or gossip or over-shopping, it is equally maddening when you cannot seem to stop yourself.

We have spent years trying to figure out how to overcome addictions and cure hidden obsessions based on the assumption that there is something on the outside of us that is causing the problem. We have examined our entire surroundings under a microscope to determine the

---

SINCE WE ARE SLAVES TO WHAT WE LOVE, IT WILL TAKE AN EVEN STRONGER LOVE TO REMOVE US.

---

root of our challenges and addictions. Billions of dollars have been spent studying the contents of cigarettes, alcohol, and food in an effort to discover what it is about them that creates in people such an inability to resist. We are constantly developing new and improved low-everything cigarettes, light beers, and fat-free foods, as well as gadgets designed to remind us to workout, limit our spending, or set time constraints on our online activity. We make the world around us change, but we do not change our hearts at all. We continue to pile our plates and fill our glasses to excess. We steadfastly wage war against pornography, yet we look longingly at our neighbor's spouse or our office co-worker. We spend endless hours and countless dollars signing up for man-made self-help seminars, yet we only learn to point the finger at others. We long for peace with God, yet we continue to look to the internet and social media for advice and approval.

We have accumulated an incredible amount of literature and established so many man-made rules, but how much have we studied our own hearts? The man-made rules dictate that we change our surroundings, but these rules have no value in changing the inside of our soul, our

---

JUST AS WE FELL IN LOVE WITH THIS STRONGHOLD, WE CAN FALL OUT OF LOVE WITH IT AND INTO A FULL, SATISFYING, AND LASTING LOVE WITH GOD.

---

inner desires. It is like treating the symptoms, but not the disease. Some over-the-counter medication works fine temporarily to get rid of a fever, but unless the correct antibiotic is given to the bacteria, it continues to exist and cause trouble. Of course, we much prefer to think that the problem lies outside ourselves so that we will not have to change, but it is simply not true. What we really need to do is reverse the focus of the heart from whatever now has our attention and our devotion over to a focus on God. Just as we fell in love with this stronghold, we can fall out of love with it and into a full, satisfying, and lasting love with God.

Colossians 2:16a, 20–23 says: Therefore do not let anyone judge you by what you eat or drink. Since you died with Christ to the basic principles of this world, why, as though you still belonged to it, do you submit to its rules: 'Do not handle! Do not taste! Do not touch!'? These are all destined to perish with use, because they are based on human commands and teachings. Such regulations indeed have an appearance of wisdom, with their self-imposed worship, their false humility and their harsh treatment of the body, but they lack any value in restraining sensual indulgence.

We have learned that it is God's will that every person seek Him and turn to Him for complete healing and freedom from man-made rules and our own strongholds. If you are new to Weigh Down, I want to assure you that you are in the right place. Weigh Down may have started as a weight loss program, but it has grown to so much more over the past three decades, helping thousands of people with all types of addictions and fixations. Weigh Down is God's way—designed by God, for God—and it is His way of living. It is about what is in your head and what is in your heart. Focus is the answer. What you focus on is everything. It is the answer for your emotional needs, your spiritual needs, your relational needs. Nothing but God can clean up your head and heart. However, there is more...down deep you have to be honest with yourself so you can tackle what is causing you pain in your life. You have turned to your stronghold or addiction for love, for comfort, for entertainment, and to take your pain away, an escape, a way to fill up your time. But here is the truth: God can do *better* than any indulgence or any addiction or any feeling you are getting from the world, hands down. Going to God is better than anything, and if you focus on God, you will fall in love with Him, and when you fall in love with Him, you will want to obey Him

---

UP TO THIS POINT, YOU HAVE SIMPLY MADE A MISTAKE BY TRYING TO FILL YOURSELF UP WITH SOMETHING FROM THIS EARTH WHEN WHAT YOU *REALLY* NEED IS A RELATIONSHIP WITH GOD!

---

more and more every day, which will lead to a life filled with blessings, contentment and joy.

In this Freedom from Strongholds Series, you will learn to recognize the difference between your normal, God-given desires and greed. Your mind will always wander to your false god. Identify it! This is the beginning of the end. Then when you feel the urge to run to that false god or that desire, instead run to God in any way you can find: take a walk, read the Bible, spend time with your spouse or children, listen to some uplifting music, send an encouraging text or call someone to lift them up, and always drop to your knees and ask for God's direction and guidance. Be sure to connect with all of the available Weigh Down resources—watch WeighDown.TV, sign up for Weigh Down social media, and visit WeighDown.com for more. It may be beneficial for you to find a friend to confide in who does not have the same stronghold you have. They may be able to help you learn the difference between what is "need" and what is "greed."

God has programmed all of us to look for a feeling in this life. Up to this point, you have simply made a mistake by trying to fill yourself up with something from this Earth when what you *really* need is a relationship with God! Take a look around you—He is everywhere! You cannot help but fall in love with Him as you begin to realize the true freedom and love He offers you. You will fall in love with what you focus on, and just as you have fallen in love with something from the world, you truly can reverse that process and fall in love with God instead. You are about to experience the fulfilling love relationship with the Almighty God for which He created you!

STRONGHOLDS

A stronghold is anything that you cling to on this Earth when God should be in its place. You depend on it, or you love it, or you worship it, or you use it for comfort, pleasure, indulgence, a high, or to feed your pride and puff yourself up. A stronghold can truly be anything on this Earth. You can make an idol of *anything*, from drugs and alcohol to sports and gambling to pornography and sexual pleasures. You can make yourself a god thru pride, anger, and gossip, or you can worship money and material objects, or you can live to gain the praise of others. Whatever your soul is seeking or whatever your mind is consuming has become your god. We all need to take a good, hard look at the inner sanctuary of our hearts—the secret places—and find out what really makes our pulse rate go up.

In the end, there will be a day when Jesus comes back for those who have made God their beginning and end—their Alpha and Omega—their all-in-all. But unfortunately, there are many individuals who have not done this. I pray for everyone, that you find God the Father thru Jesus Christ and that your soul will only feed off the true, green pasture God provides. All other feedings will not stick to the ribs and will leave your heart very empty. We must live only for eternity, not for temporary indulgences.

LIST OF STRONGHOLDS

As you look thru this list of common strongholds, let the holy, healing Spirit and personality of God reveal the special places in your heart that have not been given over fully to Him because they are filled with the perishable things on this Earth.

Substance Abuse Strongholds

- ☐ Food (eating disorders, overanalyzing, or overindulgence)
- ☐ Tobacco & Vaping
- ☐ Alcohol
- ☐ Drugs (inc. recreational marijuana)
- ☐ Overuse of Prescriptions/ Antidepressants
- ☐ Diet Pills

Emotional Strongholds

- ☐ Depression
- ☐ Self-Focused Fears
- ☐ Hate
- ☐ Jealousy
- ☐ Unworthiness/Insecurity
- ☐ Self-Focus/Self-Pity
- ☐ Hypochondria
- ☐ Protectiveness/Defensiveness

Sexual Strongholds

- ☐ Pornography
- ☐ Lewdness/Coarse Jesting or Speaking
- ☐ Sexual Lust
- ☐ Promiscuity
- ☐ Adultery

Controlling Strongholds

- ☐ Anger
- ☐ Pride/Boasting
- ☐ Credit Cards/Shopping
- ☐ Nagging
- ☐ Power/Control
- ☐ Gambling
- ☐ Greed (money, material things)
- ☐ Gossip
- ☐ Malice/Revenge
- ☐ Excessive Exercise
- ☐ Overbooked Calendar
- ☐ Anorexia/Bulimia
- ☐ Love of Money
- ☐ Overspending
- ☐ Praise from others
- ☐ Lying/Deceit
- ☐ Theft
- ☐ Social Status
- ☐ Careers
- ☐ Children (excessive focus)
- ☐ Materialism (cars, clothes, houses, etc.)
- ☐ Disrespect for Authority
- ☐ Slander
- ☐ Mocking

- ☐ Projection
- ☐ Selfish Ambition/Sabotage
- ☐ Miserliness/Stinginess
- ☐ Cursing/Profanity

Marital Strongholds

- ☐ Lack of Submission
- ☐ Misplaced Loyalty
- ☐ Marital Discord
- ☐ Selfishness
- ☐ Manipulation

Miscellaneous Strongholds

- ☐ Workaholism
- ☐ Laziness
- ☐ Procrastination
- ☐ Television/Streaming Media
- ☐ Computers/Internet

- ☐ Reality TV
- ☐ Sports (including fantasy leagues)
- ☐ Hobbies (those taking excessive attention)
- ☐ Video Games/Online Gaming
- ☐ Social Media
- ☐ Thrill Seeking
- ☐ Cooking/Recipes
- ☐ Politics/World Issues

Diagnosed Strongholds

- ☐ Hypochondria
- ☐ Anxiety
- ☐ Paranoia
- ☐ Phobias
- ☐ Personality Disorders
- ☐ Panic Attacks

The acts of the sinful nature are obvious: sexual immorality, impurity and debauchery; idolatry and witchcraft; hatred, discord, jealousy, fits of rage, selfish ambition, dissensions, factions and envy; drunkenness, orgies, and the like. I warn you, as I did before, that those who live like this will not inherit the kingdom of God.
Galatians 5:19–21

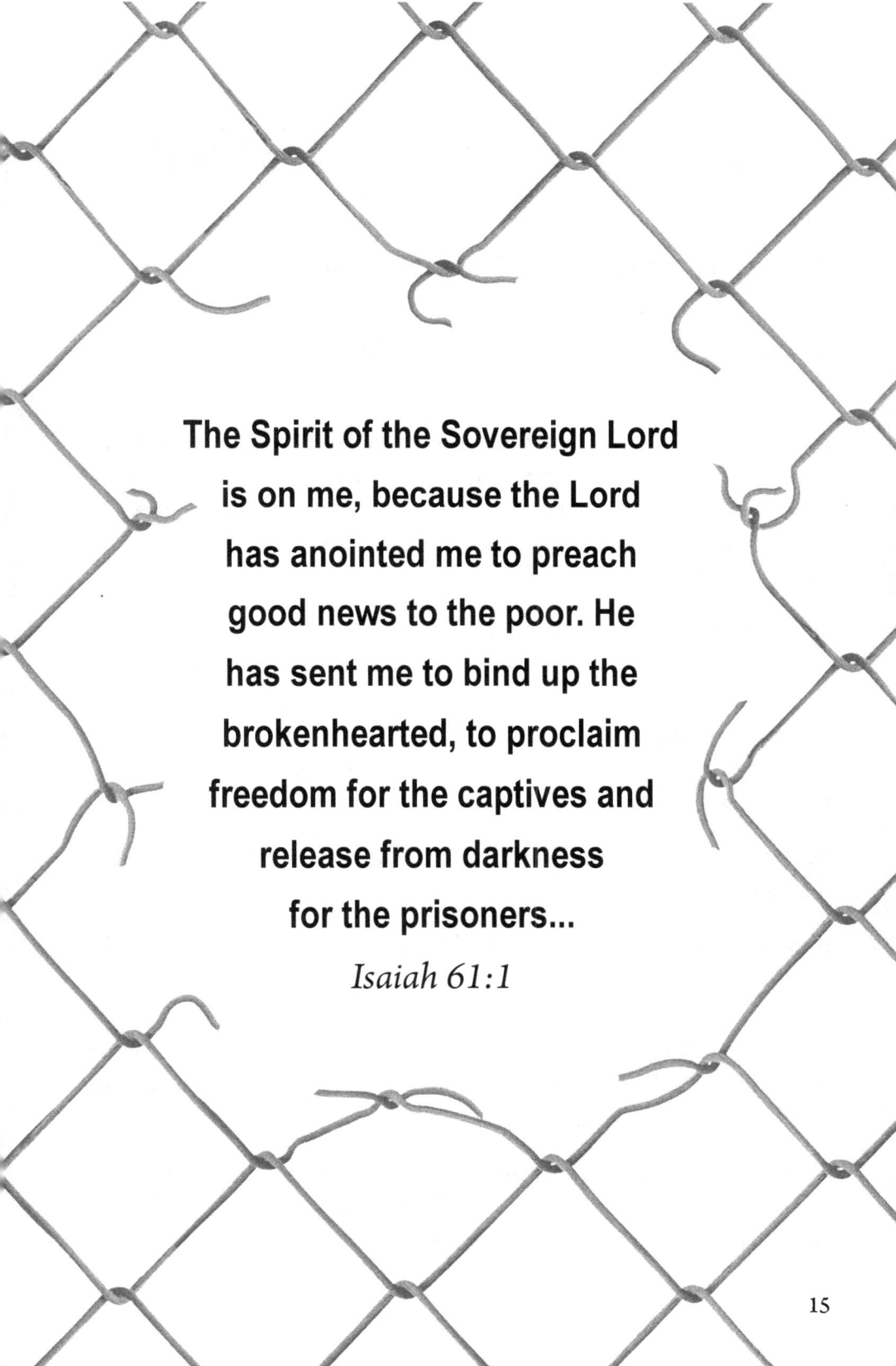

The Spirit of the Sovereign Lord is on me, because the Lord has anointed me to preach good news to the poor. He has sent me to bind up the brokenhearted, to proclaim freedom for the captives and release from darkness for the prisoners...

Isaiah 61:1

GOD IS EVERYTHING

God is...

God is my mechanic because He can fix any car, computer, or equipment.

God is my roofer. He has fixed my leaky roof without the help of human hands.

God is my husband-defender. If my husband is not present, God will act as a husband by helping me into the car with a heavy load or by protecting me when my husband is away. God lets me talk to Him when I am alone, and He meets every need, in more ways than a spouse could do.

God is my interior decorator. He can pick out colors and furniture and paintings. My whole house is a result of calling on Him for everything.

God and Christ are my best friends. Where I used to try to give someone else this position, I know thru experience that there are no friends like the Almighty God and His son, Jesus Christ.

God is my CEO for my business ventures, and the more I consult Him, the better things will go.

God is my avenger. I never think about taking revenge or getting back at someone.

God is my unsurpassed clothing consultant. He puts my outfits together in the morning. When I pray, He speeds up the decision time and great new ideas come to mind.

God is my leading party coordinator, and when I take time to pray that people have a good time, enjoy the food, and are encouraged and uplifted during the party, it is always great.

God is my only alarm clock. I have not set a real alarm clock in years, and He has always awakened me one way or another. In this way, I start talking to Him first thing every day by thanking Him for waking me up, and the rest of the day follows suit.

God is my primary songwriter and musician.

God is the journalist and Bible scholar of all my writings. I just let the Word open, and the rest is history.

God is my foremost entertainer. He always shows me something new.

God is my chief consultant for all things.

God is the great chef, and I pray over food with every meal. I want each flavor to be enjoyed and savored. Since God made everyone's taste buds, He knows exactly how to provide everyone's favorite tastes.

God is my primary physician. I go to Him in prayer first for comfort and healing. There are times God will guide me to seek out medical doctors, and I follow His lead. He created this miraculous physical body, and I do all I can to take care of His Temple.

God is my sure Savior from temptation because He has allowed Himself to be the object of my affection, not the things of this world.

God is my invisible traffic director in heavy traffic. He can part great seas of traffic, show me the best shortcuts, and provide the best parking spaces on crowded days.

God is my Everything, and when God is your Everything, you think twice about loving any other sensation on this Earth!

_____

SET FREE FROM PAIN

SCRIPTURES

- ☐ Colossians 3:1-4
- ☐ Galatians 6:7–10
- ☐ I John 1:9
- ☐ I Timothy 1:12-17
- ☐ I Peter 4:1-2
- ☐ I Peter 2:24
- ☐ Psalm 90:8
- ☐ Psalm 36:1-4
- ☐ John 8:11b
- ☐ Mark 8:34

- ☐ Isaiah 40:28-31
- ☐ Proverbs 5:7–15
- ☐ James 1:13–15
- ☐ Psalm 27:1
- ☐ Proverbs 1:20–33
- ☐ Matthew 16:23-24
- ☐ Ephesians 4
- ☐ Matthew 11:29
- ☐ I John 2:15-17
- ☐ II Peter 2:19

WEEKLY CHECKLIST

- ☐ Watch Lesson One Video
- ☐ Answer Lesson One Homework Questions
- ☐ Use your Reinforcement Resources

REINFORCEMENT RESOURCES

- ☐ *Weigh Down TV*—Watch "How to Stop Smoking"
- ☐ *Weigh Down TV*—Listen to "The Pain of the Stubborn-Hearted"
- ☐ *Weigh Down Works!*—Read the section on "Tobacco" in Chapter 20, "Alcohol, Tobacco and Drug Abuse"

THOUGHTS FROM THIS LESSON

What we have learned in this lesson is that we are free, and many of you experienced the freedom to change gods and bow down to a loving God—the freedom to take your heart, soul, mind, and strength and give them all to Jesus Christ and the heavenly Father instead of to anything on this Earth. Many of you were able to experience this freedom for the first time—no longer bowing down to your personal stronghold—and what an incredible feeling it is! What a free feeling to be able to turn off your binge-watching, to walk away from hours of online gaming, to put down the cigarette or vaping, to walk away from that refrigerator late at night, to resist that unnecessary shopping spree, to close out the adult websites, to walk away from a disagreement with no anger or rage and to feel the freedom of getting your focus OFF any nagging lust in your life!

Isn't it a wonderful opportunity to have a new boss? And our Creator is the BEST Boss! If you ever worked in a job where you had a terrible employer, then got another job under a very kind and thoughtful employer, you were overjoyed! In fact, resigning even gave you pleasure as you let the mean boss know you no longer had to endure any more stress or humiliation. At the same time, you had a new sense of purpose as you knew you were now headed in a forward direction.

You may also experience this week that the gravitational force toward the things of this world is very real. The law of sin—the greed for alcohol, food, cigarettes, drugs, power, money, and praise of mankind—is somewhat like the law of gravity in that it is real, it is powerful, it pulls you down, and it is a force that must be reckoned with. "Strongholds" are well-named. In life, if you ignore the law of gravity and walk blindly off a cliff, you will come to a premature and agonizing death. In the same way, you can ignore this reality of sin and give in to the magnetic pull of the love of worldly things and walk blindly into a premature and agonizing spiritual death.

You will become attracted to what you focus on. Your footsteps will follow your heart. If you focus on God's will, you can rise above the magnetic pull of the world. On the other hand, if you focus on the things of this world, those things will become your heartfelt desire, and that focus will lead to sin, guilt and pain.

There are two types of pain. One type of pain results from being entangled in our own sin (natural consequences), and one is pain that is screened by God and allowed by the Heavens for our own refinement. But one type of pain can end today: the pain caused by your own sin. Have you been feeling pain in your heart? You are never going to break away if you cover that pain over or try to ignore it. Start today by admitting to yourself your sins and your strongholds. Once you admit these truths to yourself, you are going to feel an immediate difference! You may feel overwhelmed at first, but you will feel instant relief as soon as you take this step, because it means you are no longer going to ignore and incubate your stronghold, but rather you are going to get it out. When you turn from sin, you will feel all the hope in the world. *If we confess our sins, he is faithful and just and will forgive us our sins and purify us from all unrighteousness. I John 1:9*

There is something so amazing about starting over. God does not want to leave you in a state of pain but rather in a state of light and joy. Praise God that sin is painful because otherwise, humans would never

---

NOTICE HOW THE MINUTE YOU FOCUS OFF THIS OBJECT OF SIN AND TURN YOUR FOCUS TO GOD AND HIS WORK, THE HURT, THE PAIN, AND THE STRESS DISAPPEAR! IT IS LIKE MAGIC.

---

look for a way out of it. Praise God there is a solution! I John 2:16 tells us clearly that being caught up in a wrong focus—the sins of the flesh, sins of the heart, sins of the eye, the pride of life—is not from the Father: *For everything in the world–the cravings of sinful man, the lust of his eyes and the boasting of what he has and does–comes not from the Father but from the world.* Notice how the minute you focus off this object of sin and turn your focus to God and His work, the hurt, the pain, and the stress disappear! It is like magic. You will feel an instant release from sin and pain, and the heavy burden will be gone. Jesus said, *"Take my yoke upon you and learn from me, for I am gentle and humble in heart, and you will find rest for your souls." Matthew 11:29*

God has a way for you to be filled with joy. It is free and instantaneous, and you can get it today. You have started the process by taking this program! It is all a choice. You only have one earthly life to live, so *therefore, since Christ suffered in his body, arm yourselves also with the same attitude, because he who has suffered in his body is done with sin. As a result, he does not live the rest of his earthly life for evil human desires, but rather for the will of God. I Peter 4:1-2* Arm yourselves with this attitude. Focus on God like you have never focused before. Feast upon the will of the Father. You can have all you want of His Spirit without ever overindulging in it!

The world talks about freedom, but who has ever heard of someone talking about the true freedom—freedom to lay down sin forever? It is available for you today, right now, to transform your mind into this attitude of Christ and accept his denial. Push away from going after money and material things. Push away from eating too much or too little. Push away from sexual sins. Push away from anger and jealousy. Push away! You are free, and you may now focus on the real freedom and shout it from the rooftops. Tell the whole world you can be done with sin right now. What are you waiting on?

You may think that your story is different, you are in too deep, your stronghold is too heavy, or your sin is too great to find this freedom we are talking about. But look at the example of the Apostle Paul! He considered himself the "worst of sinners," yet he turned immediately once his eyes were open to the opportunity to follow in Christ's example and live fully for God.[1] He did not wallow in his guilt or pain, but he was excited about this opportunity, and he was more in love with God than ever. He set his focus on the right path and did not look back.

There is no direction but one direction—end the pain of your wrong focus, accept God's mercy, and then focus your heart and mind in the right direction—on God and Christ. Then you will be truly free, free to live your life joyfully with thanksgiving, praising God and Christ for this incredible opportunity!

---

1   *See I Timothy 1:12-17.*

THOUGHT QUESTIONS

- There are several ways to find out if something is an idol. If you suspect something has become an idol in your life, remove it. Let it be taken away and see what is revealed in your heart. For example, if you suspect you are addicted to alcohol, try to go a whole week without a drink. If it is pornography, attempt an entire month without visiting any questionable websites or apps. If it is tobacco or vaping, throw away all the tobacco, e-cigarettes, or vaping cartridges in the house and see how that affects you over the coming days. If it is food, try to wait until you are physiologically hungry until you pick up that snack, or cut your regular meal amounts down and see if that amount satisfies you. If you suspect you are obsessed with gossip, try not to talk about anyone in a gossipy way for a whole week. If you worry that you might be addicted to your phone or to social media, set real boundaries for using your apps and social media in the coming month and see how you do. (See the list of possible strongholds on page 13.)

  We were all born to love and to worship something. The fact is, you can make anything on this Earth an idol if you find yourself loving it to a fault. Before you know it, you might even find yourself enslaved to several things at one time—for instance, sexual lust, alcohol, gaming, and money. In fact, when you looked over the list of strongholds in the Introduction, you were probably surprised at how many of those areas have a hold on your heart and your focus! If you long for something, you know that your heart has been given over to that stronghold. Another way to identify an idol is to examine what you worry about or what your mind wanders to all day long. II Peter 2:19 says that a man is a slave to whatever has mastered him. Spend some time today with God and identify what you are longing for or worrying about, what is causing your lack of peace and contentment. Ask God to reveal to you the strongholds He wants you to give up. Be completely honest with yourself and with God. Record those strongholds here and ask Him to lead you out of this prison so that you can love Him fully!

_____

_____

_____

_____

_____

- *So I tell you this, and insist on it in the Lord, that you must no longer live as the Gentiles do, in the futility of their thinking. They are darkened in their understanding and separated from the life of God because of the ignorance that is in them due to the hardening of their hearts. Having lost all sensitivity, they have given themselves over to sensuality so as to indulge in every kind of impurity, with a continual lust for more. You, however, did not come to know Christ that way. Surely you heard of him and were taught in him in accordance with the truth that is in Jesus. You were taught, with regard to your former way of life, to put off your old self, which is being corrupted by its deceitful desires; to be made new in the attitude of your minds; and to put on the new self, created to be like God in true righteousness and holiness. Ephesians 4:17–24* According to this passage, God is calling us to a new life, and obviously, the early Christians had the same struggle. Please read the entire chapter of Ephesians 4 and list the ways we are to be pure-hearted.

_____

_____

_____

_____

_____

- Think about the effects of your stronghold on your life. How has it imprisoned you? For example—if you are overweight, the added heaviness may have caused discomfort, bone and joint problems, sleeping problems, etc. If you are addicted to alcohol, it has probably harmed your relationships with family and friends, caused embarrassment, and maybe even brought about expensive legal issues. If you are in love with money or material possessions, you may be imprisoned in a workaholic state, obsessed with gambling and easy-money schemes, or left in a state of bankruptcy. List below how your strongholds have affected you:

_____

_____

_____

_____

_____

- Read Colossians 2:16–23 again (see page 6). Describe some of the man-made approaches that you have used in trying to overcome your stronghold (such as setting restrictions to limit computer or app time, attending specialized support groups, applying nicotine patches, switching to light beer, avoiding social situations where your stronghold would be present, etc.).

_____

_____

_____

_____

_____

_____

_____

- Even though some man-made approaches might restrict your ability to obtain those strongholds, have any of these approaches made your heart desire that stronghold any less?

  _____

  _____

  _____

  _____

  _____

  _____

- According to the verse you just read (Colossians 2:16–23) and what you have learned so far, why do you think these methods have failed to help you make permanent changes?

  _____

  _____

  _____

  _____

  _____

- Changing your focus—your mindset—is crucial in breaking free from a stronghold. _Those who live according to the sinful nature have their minds set on what that nature desires; but those who live in accordance with the Spirit have their minds set on what the Spirit desires. The mind of sinful man is death, but the mind controlled by the Spirit is life and peace; the sinful mind is hostile to God. It does not submit to God's law, nor can it do so. Those controlled by the sinful nature cannot please God._ Romans 8:5–8

  The word "focus" is used frequently in this Series. Read Colossians 3:1–4, Galatians 6:7–10, and Philippians 4:8. What do these scriptures ask us to focus on?

_____

_____

_____

_____

• List some specific things that you can now focus on instead of your old focus. Compare these notes with other class members or online encouragement friends.

_____

_____

_____

_____

_____

• The following scriptures all convey one main thought. Let's start with Galatians 5:16–25: *So I say, live by the Spirit, and you will not gratify the desires of the sinful nature. For the sinful nature desires what is contrary to the Spirit, and the Spirit what is contrary to the sinful nature. They are in conflict with each other, so that you do not do what you want. But if you are led by the Spirit, you are not under law. The acts of the sinful nature are obvious: sexual immorality, impurity and debauchery; idolatry and witchcraft; hatred, discord, jealousy, fits of rage, selfish ambition, dissensions, factions and envy; drunkenness, orgies, and the like. I warn you, as I did before, that those who live like this will not inherit the kingdom of God. But the fruit of the Spirit is love, joy, peace, patience, kindness, goodness, faithfulness, gentleness and self-control. Against such things there is no law. Those who belong to Christ Jesus have crucified the sinful nature with its passions and desires. Since we live by the Spirit, let us keep in step with the Spirit.*

Now read Ephesians 4:17-24, Colossians 3:1–11, 1 John 3:1–10, 1 John 2:3–6, and 2 Peter 2:4–22. All these passages convey one main idea. Summarize that idea below.

_____

_____

_____

_____

_____

- Spend some serious time thinking about and recounting any way your stronghold has helped you, comforted you, filled your heart, strengthened you, or given back to you. Then think about all the ways that stronghold has harmed you and robbed you spiritually, financially, relationally, and physically. Refer back to these lists every time you feel a craving for your stronghold.

  Rewards of idols:

  _____

  _____

  _____

  Consequences of idols:

  _____

  _____

  _____

  _____

  _____

- Think about how often your mind wanders to your secret love or your heart craves your secret stronghold and record the number of times each day you are having to battle temptation. In addition, record the specific times of day or specific situations when these temptations seem to be worse. Recognizing these battles means you are recognizing the pull of your stronghold and fighting against it! Acknowledging your more difficult times of temptation will help you become more battle-ready so you can make changes to help you be victorious during these times.

How many times do you battle temptation each day? _____

What times of the day or situations are the hardest when it comes to being tempted by your strongholds?

_____

_____

_____

What kinds of things can you do to be battle-ready during these times?

_____

_____

_____

• If you stay focused on God, these moments of temptation should happen less and less frequently as the weeks go by. In a few weeks, come back to this page and compare this number and notice your progress! These battles will soon be less intense, and as time passes, you will only have occasional temptations that do not have the intensity of these battles. The fire will die out if you do not fan the flame. Make sure you are making this journey a daily priority in your life, for nothing is more important than learning to love God with all of your heart, all of your mind, all of your soul, and all of your strength.

LESSON 1 HOMEWORK ASSIGNMENT

Find someone this week—a friend, co-worker, family member—who is not magnetized to your particular stronghold and watch how they react around it. For example, if your stronghold is overindulgence in alcohol, watch the behavior of a moderate drinker and how they approach alcohol. If your addiction is food and overeating, watch how someone without this struggle approaches a meal or snacks. If you are battling sexual lust, find someone who has, like Job, made a covenant with their eyes to not look lustfully at another person.[1] Talk to these people and ask them *why* they would never overindulge, overeat, or cheat on their spouse. What is their motivation?

_____

_____

_____

_____

_____

_____

_____

_____

_____

_____

_____

_____

_____

_____

_____

_____

---

1   *I made a covenant with my eyes not to look lustfully at a girl. Job 31:1*

COUNTING YOUR BLESSINGS

Recognizing the countless blessings God has given you will be so important on this journey! Recount all the ways that God has blessed you, given to you, cared for you, and helped you. The more you fill in this list every day, the less magnetized you will be toward your stronghold. Spend extra time on your knees and on your face in prayer before the Father. Cry out to God and praise Him for letting you find Him and talk directly to Him. Think about it—it is so difficult to get close to famous people, yet here is the richest, most famous, most talented, and most well-known Being in the Universe, and He wants to hear from you, and He longs to have your love. Praise God for allowing you to get close to Him! Focus this week on the heavenly Father and Jesus Christ, and you will have a great week as you learn to approach each day, minute by minute, hour by hour! (Note: This question will be repeated each week)

Example: God, thank you for letting me live today. I was able to share the day with my friends and family! I know you give life, and I know you take it away, so I am thankful for today! Thank you for Jesus Christ who died so that we may live in a rewarding relationship forever. Jesus, praise your name for this supreme love and for your ultimate example of "Not my will, but Yours be done." Luke 22:42. You might have preferred it to just be you and God in Heaven, but due to your ultimate sacrifice, you have allowed us to personally draw near to God as well, and for this we are eternally grateful.

_____

_____

_____

_____

COMMON STRUGGLE FOR LESSON 1

You will encounter struggles as you work your way thru this 8-lesson Series. This is perfectly normal and part of God's plan in order that this life-changing material will be planted deeply into your heart. The main struggle of Lesson One is understanding the concept of recognizing and admitting your own strongholds and learning how to start breaking away from them. It is a new concept to realize there is nothing wrong with the created things on this Earth and admitting that the whole problem lies within our own hearts–the greed we have allowed to grow for those things and our reliance and dependence upon them for feelings or comfort.

Read Mark 7:14–23 and I Timothy 4:1-4. Remember that this is a journey for your heart, and you do not have to be a scholar. No one is going to be looking over your shoulder, and you do not have to fill in everything in the workbook to be successful. There is no formula to this, and there is no legalism. If some of the concepts are not sinking in today, remember that we will be going over these ideas and scriptures again and again until they sink into your heart. Our suggestion is to find someone else who is taking this program, either online or in person, who seems to be excited about this journey and is putting it into practice, and spend some time chatting, texting, and encouraging one another. Overall, please do not worry. This is more of a love story seminar than a spiritual marathon. Relax and enjoy learning how much the Father adores you!

PRAYER

Dear God, help us all to be blind to the strongholds of this world and open our eyes to seek only you. Thank you for your personal love and caring in allowing us to experience pain when we have the wrong focus, yet experience beautiful jewels and blessings when we focus our heart, soul, mind, and strength on You! Amen.

LESSON 2

GOD'S BOUNDARIES

SCRIPTURES

- [ ] Proverbs 8:27-29
- [ ] Psalm 74:16-17
- [ ] Deuteronomy 8:1-3
- [ ] Psalm 16:5-8
- [ ] Isaiah 26: 1-4
- [ ] II Thessalonians 3:6–13
- [ ] John 14:15–24a
- [ ] Proverbs 15:17–18
- [ ] Proverbs 10:4

- [ ] Luke 12:13–21
- [ ] Proverbs 11:2
- [ ] Proverbs 23:1–3
- [ ] Philippians 3:17–21
- [ ] Deuteronomy 30:19-20
- [ ] Titus 2:3, 11-14
- [ ] Proverbs 20:1
- [ ] Proverbs 21:17
- [ ] Ephesians 5:18

WEEKLY CHECKLIST

- [ ] Watch Lesson Two Video
- [ ] Answer Lesson Two Homework Questions
- [ ] Use your Reinforcement Resources

REINFORCEMENT RESOURCES

- [ ] *Weigh Down TV*—Watch "How to Change Your Life in 30 Days"
- [ ] *Weigh Down TV*—Watch "How to Be Free from Alcohol Addictions"
- [ ] *Weigh Down Works!*—Read the section on "Alcohol" in Chapter 20, "Alcohol, Tobacco and Drug Abuse"

THOUGHTS FROM THIS LESSON

Welcome to Lesson Two of breaking away from your strongholds! You have hopefully had a few days of tasting freedom since you started this Series, and you are moving further and further away from the things of this world…and more importantly, are feeling yourself moving nearer and nearer to God! You have probably won some battles and lost some battles, but you are learning so much about your heart! Now, as you become more and more aware of how vigorously your strongholds call you back, you will begin to enter what we refer to as the Desert of Testing.

The first few days of this program gave you a fresh start and the hope of a new freedom, aided by a focus on God. This focus on God led you out of your prison and into an exciting independence from your particular stronghold. Some of you laid down anger and control. Some experienced fewer panic attacks and less worry. Some had no episodes of bulimia. Others put down their credit cards or their e-cigarettes, their overdrinking or recreational drugs. Some set aside their pride and their controlling nature and replaced that with humility, and their jobs and marriages seemed better this week. Some have experienced several days in a row with no sexual temptations and have been filled with inexpressible joy that they are now free to love God and put down those guilt-ridden lusts. Whatever strongholds God is calling you to let go of seemed to have much less control over you the past week!

You may notice that now you feel a little different. That is because you are starting to enter the Desert of Testing. Deuteronomy 8:1–3 says: *Be careful to follow every command I am giving you today, so that you may live and increase and may enter and possess the land that the lord promised on oath to your forefathers. Remember how the lord your God led you all the way in the desert these forty years, to humble you and to test you in order to know what was in your heart, whether or not you would keep his commands. He humbled you, causing you to hunger and then feeding you with manna, which neither you nor your fathers had known, to teach you that man does not live on bread alone but on every word that comes from the mouth of the Lord.*

God is taking you to a place where there is not one piece of the world to flirt with your attention. The desert is barren, dry, and lifeless, and the only way that you can survive is to quickly find the Water and the Shade—God Almighty and Jesus Christ. Their words will be your flashlight in the dark and the water you need to make it thru a dry, thirsty land. God has heard your decision to follow Him fully instead of giving your heart to idols, but now this decision must drop down into the heart.

In the Biblical story in the book of Exodus, God showed His mighty power and used Moses to lead the Hebrews away from the slavery of Egypt into the freedom to worship God alone. God even parted the Red Sea to separate the Israelites fully away from the land of idols, and He led them into the hot, dry desert for the next forty years. This desert was a place where He was able to test their hearts, to see if their devotion was true and real, and to see if they would be tempted to return to the slavery of Egypt. It is also the place where God presented them with their new Law, the Ten Commandments, of which the very first commandment was that there should be no idols before Him in their hearts or minds.

The desert is the place to fall in love with God and out of love with the false idols. Your newly entered spiritual desert will serve the same purpose. As we have stated earlier, we must start by exposing this false attraction, addiction, or false god. Has this stronghold helped your finances? No, it has robbed you. All addictions are expensive. Even if the acquisition of money is your idol, there is no real joy in that because you will find you never have enough. Has your stronghold helped with your self-esteem? No. Has your idol helped with your relationships? No—it has put a wedge between you and your spouse or family members. Has your idol helped with your health? No—it has taken your sleep, your physical well-being, your peace of mind, and sometimes even caused irreparable physical damage. This false god turns out to be a parasitic leech that robs you of your time, passion, money, devotion, peace, and self-esteem. It is a false master—a false lover leaving you with only unrequited love. It is a false friend. It offers only a temporary pleasure that leaves you with increasing troubles, guilt, emotional deprivation, and physical ailments. There is a very high price to pay for grabbing at a worldly passion instead of letting God fill you up!

Here is a challenge for you, to help you see a difference between your idol and the One True God! God keeps on proving that He is God, and we have forgotten what a true God is. Take 10 minutes that you would have spent on your stronghold and give it to God. Instead of sitting on the sofa and playing yet another round of a video game, ask God how He would rather you spend your time—maybe in prayer, maybe working on this workbook or reading a Bible chapter, maybe calling a friend or family member who needs encouragement. A true God does not "need" your 10 minutes, so He will give you back an hour, and you will suddenly find that you have more time in your day! He does not need your money—He is a true God and needs nothing. So try this: take the 10 dollars you would have spent on that stronghold and give

---

INSIDE GOD'S BOUNDARIES IS TRUE PEACE AND JOY AND ALL THAT YOU COULD EVER WANT OR NEED.

---

it to God. You can donate it to church or to a local charity; you can use it on a sweet, unexpected gift for a friend or family member who needs encouragement; you can use it to pay off debt instead of increasing your debts, etc. He will multiply it and give you back blessings! You see, God does not need your time or your money. However, because you freely gave it to Him and because He truly loves you, He takes your gift and offers it back in multiples!

God has it all and is very generous to hearts that love Him. You may not believe He really is there and is that personal, but just try it. If you run to Him for everything, you will be in for a big surprise. The rewards and jewels will be there—just look for them. Running to God for comfort and solutions makes sense, while running to your idols for comfort and solutions makes no sense at all. God's Word is a true light unto your path. What would be wrong with having more reverence, more attention, more emotion, more passion, more love for God? Love always grows, and you want to make sure your love is growing for God, not for your stronghold. The fact is, whatever you are focused on, you will be more in love with that next year. So where is your focus? A year from now, will you be more in love with God…or with your stronghold? How could you not want your growing focus to be on something glorious and beautiful? What are you looking at and focusing on this very day? This very hour? If it is an idol or stronghold, it pales in comparison to God Almighty.

A lot of times people give God their day, but then they do not give Him their night. You have to be still and open your eyes to really see how you are spending your time throughout the whole day. Keep in mind that you cannot see clearly until you have laid down the stronghold, because until you lay down your sin, all that sparkles for you will be your refrigerator or your adult websites or your alcohol. Maybe your sight is clouded by materialism or your love of money. Maybe what pulls your attention is indulging yourself, scrolling mindless social media, or spreading the latest gossip. Maybe you are being blinded to Truth by the anticipation of the next drink, the next vape, the next sexual thrill. These are all things developed by the Creator to be used correctly (with no greed beyond His boundaries) when we are living life totally devoted to Him. God's boundaries are so important! For your hands to dip into God's pockets and grab for more than what He has given you is totally self-focused, spoiled, immoral, and embarrassing.

The boundary lines have fallen for me in pleasant places. Psalm 16:6 Those who are miserable in life are those who are consistently trying to step beyond God's boundaries. What is it that you want for your own child or grandchild? Do you not want them to be temperate, to be content, to have no anger? Do you not want them to be happy inside God's boundaries? Do you want to pass down your secret sins or addictions or strongholds? Inside God's boundaries is true peace and joy and all that you could ever want or need…as the scripture above states, God's boundary lines fall in pleasant places. It is your own greed and idolatry that do not like the boundary lines, but outside God's boundary lines, there is only discontent, destruction, and spiritual (sometimes even physical) death.

People think they can keep stepping across the boundary lines and face no consequences. Some over-drinkers boldly think they will not destroy their liver, but alcohol is an extremely demanding molecule. In the liver–the chemical factory where all this occurs–the alcohol will demand to be completely broken down first, thereby pushing back the breaking down of fats and sugars. So the fats remain in the system, waiting to be mobilized. When the alcohol finally gets broken down, it is also turned into a fat. The triglycerides then land into the liver and sit there, like at a bus stop, also waiting to be broken down. If all this cannot be broken down, it will simply keep accumulating. After some time, that immobile fat will harden, and when it hardens, it prevents circulation in the liver. This is basically a slow death to the liver. It can make you very ill, and in many cases, it can lead to death.

That happens over time, but drinking in excess in even a single setting can also be very detrimental. There are many stories of young adults binge drinking or putting themselves in dangerous situations–even resulting in death–from playing around with alcohol. There are also countless deaths due to alcohol poisoning, where the body simply cannot process the overabundance of alcohol someone is putting into it. God designed our bodies to try and stay healthy, and most people can identify cues from the body that it does not like the feeling of overdrinking! There are very clear indications that you have gone beyond God's boundaries if you feel the least bit ill or experience any of God's warning signs He incorporated into our physical system. The good news is that the body wants to be healthy; it wants to reverse this process…so how do you do it? How do you reverse the damage done by stepping outside God's boundaries with alcohol? Just put it down. Lay off it. Fast from the alcohol and leave it behind for a while. Let it clear out of your system. Allow the liver to heal. Thru all this, ask for God's Spirit, because God does not overdrink! That is not His personality!

What about tobacco use or vaping? Countless scientific studies show that smoking tobacco, using e-cigarettes, and vaping can be very dangerous and damaging to the body. Even secondary smoke has been shown to cause cancer in the body. If you recall, when you were a child, your body did not like having to breathe in smoke or strange vapor. No child ever says, "I want to go into a smoky room" or "Let the fireplace smoke up the house. This is awesome!" To the contrary, your body says, "No–breathing in this smoke does not feel good!" In addition, many people are allergic to smoke or vapor or have asthma; breathing in smoke or vapor can cause headaches and breathing problems, because the body desperately wants to get away and find fresh air. Besides the lung problems that breathing in smoke or vapor can cause, the chemicals contained in tobacco products or vaping products have been shown to cause serious physical consequences. The addiction to nicotine spans across all forms of tobacco and e-cigarette use, and sadly, with vaping, these problems are affecting even younger and younger ages.

Today, you are starting over! You will be living each day for God's holy, incredibly temperate Spirit. With that Spirit, you can have a drink and not overdrink. You can enjoy a meal and not binge. You can shop online and stay within a budget. You can attend an event with your spouse and not let your eye and your lust wander to other people. You can check social media on your phone, then put your phone down instead of losing the next three hours to it. You can work online and not be tempted to click over to adult websites. You can spend an entire day with your family and not nag them, control them with anger or passive aggressiveness, or try to manipulate them. You can enjoy coffee with your friends and not gossip or slander others. The peace and content- ment that will come into your heart will be so much more filling than any of your strongholds! You are about to experience what being Spirit- led feels like!

When you bypass all God's signals over and over, you are willfully bypassing His boundaries, and that will never be fruitful. Think for a moment…what sea would do that to God, constantly flowing outside its boundaries, ruining the shoreline, killing people, destroying homes, making marshes everywhere that God never intended a marsh? What wind would do that to God, continually blowing with such force that trees are stripped, landscapes are decimated, homes and cities are ruined, and no crops can grow? The sea moves and the wind blows as God intends, for there is no other way.

You can do this, too! Consider God's boundaries as precious and untouchable. When there is something offered or a situation that presents itself that is beyond God's boundary for you, you say "No" and you remove yourself from the situation if possible. When you say "No" to this temptation, it begins to die. And then the next time, you say again, "No, I do not want to go beyond His boundaries," and the draw of the temptation dies a little more. If you think you cannot do this, read Titus 2:11-14: *For the grace of God that brings salvation has appeared to all men. It teaches us to say "No" to ungodliness and worldly passions, and to live self-controlled, upright and godly lives in this present age, while we wait for the blessed hope—the glorious appearing of our great God and Savior, Jesus Christ, who gave himself for us to redeem us from all wickedness and to purify for himself a people that are his very own, eager to do what is good.*

You CAN do this, for this is God's plan for you! You CAN be a person who belongs to Him alone, eager to do what is good, not eager to cross His boundaries and then suffer the pain that comes with it! When you are tempted, say "No" to ungodliness. Turn away. Suffer it away. Fast from the sin. Let it go. When you are truly done with the suffering, you will be done with the sin...and what freedom that will be, to no longer even experience those temptations! *He who has suffered in his body is done with sin and therefore no longer lives the rest of his earthly life for his own evil desires but rather for the will of God. I Peter 4:1-2*

It is time to show God that you truly want to put Him first. You are entering the Desert of Testing. The testing might get hot as you continue to turn away from your temptations, but do not give up! The heat of the desert and the refining that will come from this experience is so much better than the pain of the consequences you feel when you cross over God's boundaries. This is such a sweet time; how fun is that time of your life when you are living for God, in step with His Spirit, listening for and hearing His voice! When you love Him fully, your focus will be on Him—not your strongholds anymore—and you will not even be tempted to go beyond what He has sweetly and generously provided for you. Trust in the Lord your God! He has provided beautiful boundaries for you individually. He is so personal, and remember what we read above: His boundaries have fallen in pleasant places, and look what it leads to! *The boundary lines have fallen for me in pleasant places; surely I have a delightful inheritance. Psalm 16:6*

A delightful inheritance! So starting today, reverse your past behavior and no longer obey the temptations or lusts or alluring call of the things of this world. No longer brag about, revel in, or make light of your idols or your strongholds. Instead, obey and long for and brag about the Father! Say "no" to worldly cravings and temptations and "yes" to your loving Father. True love will be returned to you in special and personal ways that could only come from Him; it will be undeniable. Thru obedience and blessings, you will continue to fall more in love with God.

THOUGHT QUESTIONS

- Ask God to help you identify someone who is wholeheartedly and joyfully in love with the Father—someone who has no secret idols or temptations. Try to get to know them and pray with them and imitate them. Watch how their eyes light up when you ask them about what God did for them that week and what He taught them. Watch their excitement as they find out that you are interested in talking about their passion! It will be like the old feeling of finding a drinking buddy or golf buddy or gossip buddy. Spend time finding out how they fell in love with God more than anything on the Earth and record their story here.

_____

_____

_____

_____

_____

_____

- Spend some additional time this week recounting all the pain that your false comforts and idols have caused you and your family, friends, and coworkers. List these here so you can see what you will be leaving behind to live for God!

  _____

  _____

  _____

  _____

  _____

  _____

- In this lesson, you were asked to try taking 10 minutes that you would have spent on your idol and giving that time to God instead. Try that today and record here how God gives back!

  _____

  _____

- Read the passages below and record what happens if you worship the following strongholds:

  Anger/hatred—Proverbs 15:17–18, I John 2:9, Ephesians 4:31

  _____

  _____

  Laziness/idleness—Proverbs 10:4 and 2 Thessalonians 3:6–13

  _____

  _____

  Love of money—Job 31:24–28, Luke 12:13–21 and Ecclesiastes 5:10–20

  _____

  _____

The praise of man or pride—Proverbs 11:2, Proverbs 29:23, 15:25, 16:19

_____

_____

Love of food or gluttony—Proverbs 23:1–3 and Philippians 3:17–21

_____

_____

Alcohol abuse—Isaiah 5:11, Proverbs 23:29–35 and 21:17

_____

_____

Drug dependence/substance abuse—I Peter 4:7 and 5:8, Romans 12:1

_____

_____

Judgmentalism—Matthew 7:1–5 and James 2:12

_____

_____

Sexual lust—Proverbs 5, Job 31:9–12, and Matthew 5:27–28

_____

_____

Theft—Ephesians 4:28, Proverbs 20:23 and Proverbs 21:6

_____

_____

Foolish talk/gossip—Ephesians 5:3–7, Proverbs 12:13, 16:28, and 18:21

_____

_____

Greed—Proverbs 15:27, Haggai 1:5-6

_____

_____

- Now look up the following scriptures and contrast what happens if you come to the True God for comfort, joy, help, defense, direction, and life.

  ☐ Isaiah 54:11–17   ☐ Proverbs 16:7
  ☐ Isaiah 58:6–12   ☐ Proverbs 21:21
  ☐ Proverbs 11:16   ☐ Psalm 103
  ☐ Proverbs 11:25   ☐ Psalm 112
  ☐ Proverbs 16:3   ☐ Deuteronomy 28:1-14

  _____

  _____

  _____

- You have probably heard of behavior modification. The general principle is that when you do right, you are praised and rewarded so that you will repeat that good behavior. If you do wrong, you have consequences so that you will not repeat that behavior. This is referred to as behavior modification, and God obviously wants our behavior modified or He would not have set up this system of punishment and rewards from the very beginning. Look up Deuteronomy 28 and record the blessings we can expect for doing right and the curses we can expect for doing wrong.

Blessings:

_____

_____

Curses:

_____

_____

- God is the great Behavior Modification Specialist, and He is working hard to wake you up, because He disciplines those whom He loves, and He wants you to realize how much He truly loves you. Read Hebrews 12:5-11 about God's love and His discipline. According to this passage, whom does God discipline? What does God's discipline produce in us?

_____

_____

- Think about the ways God has shown you His positive rewards in recent days as you have been committed to seeking Him. Write down your victories (no matter how small!) and His rewards, blessings, and answered prayers as you took your mind off your stronghold and overcame its magnetic pull.

Victories:

_____

_____

_____

Rewards:

_____

_____

- As you go thru this Series, use the following worksheet from *Weigh Down Works!* to help track your progress as you transfer your focus off of your stronghold and onto God!

WEIGHDOWN DEPENDENCIES WORKSHEET

Did you go outside of God's will today with your dependency?	❏ Yes ❏ No
Did you PRAY when the temptation came up? Did you run to the Word of God?	❏ Yes ❏ No
Did you AT LEAST set your clock to "20 minutes" to see if—by prayer—a way of escape would come from God?	❏ Yes ❏ No
When temptation for your dependency came up, did you "flip" the lies from satan and quote the TRUTH?	❏ Yes ❏ No
How many tests with your dependency did you pass today?	
How many did you fail?	
Do you feel you spent more time TRANSFER-RING your focus to GOD today instead of focusing on your dependency?	❏ Yes ❏ No
Do you feel more READY and PREPARED to obey God's voice over the voice from your dependency?	❏ Yes ❏ No
Do you feel your heart improving toward more of a love for God?	❏ Yes ❏ No
Write down the number of times you messed up. (*Complete this worksheet daily for one month, and watch the number go down. See WeighDown.com for more copies.*)	

WeighDown © 2014 by Gwen Shamblin and WeighDown Ministries. www.WeighDown.com

COMMON STRUGGLE FOR LESSON 2

You are entering the Desert of Testing. God is moving you away from your idol and into a dry desert where it will just be you and Him. At first, breaking away from your stronghold might have seemed easier because of the excitement of this new freedom, but you may begin to really feel the pain of separation from your stronghold this week. The good news is that this testing will be short-lived if you stay focused on the Father. If you have still been unable to make a transfer of your focus off the stronghold and onto God, it is because you have only mentally recognized that God is the one true God to worship, and you have only mentally acknowledged that you should let go of this worldly lusting. It is time to wake up your heart, and you can do that thru recognizing and fully obeying God's boundaries... not just making a mental acknowledgement, but putting this new focus into practice. Drop everything distracting that is going on in your life and fully respect God's boundaries each day with regard to your strongholds. Once you do this, you will experience letting God provide the very best for you, better than you could have imagined for yourself! Pray over every aspect, every moment, every temptation, and every success. After all, if you ask, you will receive.[1] But if you do not ask, you will not receive. Go to God with everything during this Desert of Testing, and you will be rewarded. He is so much better than giving in to any cravings and temptations of the world!

PRAYER

Dear Heavenly Father, help me to recognize your perfect boundaries for my life, and help me to experience pure obedience to those boundaries. Help me not to be afraid to let go of my strongholds so that I may experience what you have to offer, because I know it will be so much better! Wake up my heart to your amazing love, and help me permanently close the doors to my old strongholds. Amen.

---

1   *Ask and it will be given to you; seek and you will find; knock and the door will be opened to you. For everyone who asks receives; he who seeks finds; and to him who knocks, the door will be opened. Matthew 7:7-8*

COUNTING YOUR BLESSINGS

Recognizing the countless blessings God has given you will be so important on this journey! Recount all the ways that God has blessed you, given to you, cared for you, and helped you. The more you fill in this list every day, the less magnetized you will be toward your stronghold. Spend extra time on your knees and on your face in prayer before the Father. Cry out to God and praise Him for letting you find Him and talk directly to Him. Think about it—it is so difficult to get close to famous people… yet here is the richest, most famous, most talented, and most well-known Being in the Universe, and He wants to hear from you, and He longs to have your love. Praise God for allowing you to get close to Him! Focus this week on the heavenly Father and Jesus Christ, and you will have a great week as you learn to approach each day, minute by minute, hour by hour!

Example: Dear God, praise you for allowing us to worship you every day. May we always appreciate the opportunity to learn about you, to freely talk about you and pray to you. May we never forget that when two or three are gathered together, you are willing to come into our midst, so thank you for the fellow sojourners who are experiencing this journey with me. I am not alone, so thank you for the friendships that are based on loving you first. May we never take lightly that we are able to have the richest, most powerful, most intelligent Leader of the Universe taking care of us, guiding us, and providing such pleasant and peaceful boundaries for us. We have it all and do not want to take that for granted. Open our eyes, Lord, and let us truly show our thankfulness by choosing you over any stronghold. In Jesus' name, Amen.

_____
_____
_____
_____
_____
_____
_____
_____
_____
_____
_____
_____
_____
_____
_____
_____
_____
_____
_____
_____
_____
_____
_____
_____
_____
_____

CLEAR-MINDED AND SELF-CONTROLLED

SCRIPTURES

- [ ] I Corinthians 10:13
- [ ] Exodus 34:14
- [ ] John 15:7
- [ ] John 4:10-13
- [ ] Jeremiah 17:9
- [ ] Matthew 6:24
- [ ] Luke 8:4–15
- [ ] I Peter 5:8-9
- [ ] I Peter 4:7
- [ ] Romans 12:1
- [ ] Romans 13:1

- [ ] I Chronicles 28:9
- [ ] Matthew 7:9–11
- [ ] I Samuel 2:8
- [ ] Ephesians 6:6–7
- [ ] I John 4:20
- [ ] Philippians 2:12
- [ ] Psalm 143:8
- [ ] II Corinthians 10:3–5
- [ ] Luke 18:18–27
- [ ] Jonah 2:8

WEEKLY CHECKLIST

- [ ] Watch Lesson Three Video
- [ ] Answer Lesson Three Homework Questions
- [ ] Use your Reinforcement Resources

REINFORCEMENT RESOURCES

- [ ] *Weigh Down TV*—Listen to "Save Your Heart for Me"
- [ ] *Weigh Down TV*—Watch "How To Be Transformed—Displacement and Meditation"
- [ ] *Weigh Down Works!*—Read the section on "Illicit Drugs" in Chapter 20, "Alcohol, Tobacco and Drug Abuse"
- [ ] *History of the Love of God*—Read Chapter 27, "Greater Love has No One"

THOUGHTS FROM THIS LESSON

In this lesson, we learned that any relationship, any love for another, is reciprocal and based on "give and take." Denying self is just another way of giving. The more you deny yourself, the less you will actually start to desire...and your stronghold will have less and less pull on you. This new self-control you will discover is a gift straight from God's Holy Spirit! You will find that the more you give of yourself and your own selfish desires, the more you are able to break free from the earthly desires of drugs, money, lust, food, and any other strongholds. Less is more and more is less; God's Spirit is a compelling, life-transforming power that gives back everything and fills your heart and soul.

Denial is an essential part of our relationships here on this Earth. When someone does something for you, what feeling does that bring forth in you? You trust that person, you have no fear, you have peace. Denial of self will bring about gentleness and closeness with others. But be aware that the opposite is also true—if you stop denying self and giving and you fall back into selfishness and self-focus, the closeness will begin to fade and your relationships with your spouse, children, and friends will suffer. The old greed will rise up again, and once it starts growing again, it will set off a continual lust for more.

We must stop "playing God" in our lives. We are not a god. Ezekiel 28:2 is very clear about this! The mindset of being your own god will ruin everything our True God is trying to establish. Do you want to be above God? Or do you want a real relationship with God? You cannot have it both ways...make a choice today and commit to living it out! Start over this very minute. Satan tries to make "denial" so overwhelming and scary...but again, it is just the opposite. You will be so blessed in all areas if you build this relationship where God is your true God. Sacrifice your own selfish desires, deny yourself the things that are outside of God's boundaries, and live for Him. In doing so, you will discover amazing peace and contentment and love.

And God is right there with you to help you when you are tested. I Corinthians 10:13 says, *No temptation has seized you except what is common to man. And God is faithful; He will not let you be tempted beyond what you can bear. But when you are tempted, He will provide a way out so that you can stand up under it.* On this journey away from our strong-holds, we take this verse literally...God Himself will devise a way for us out of a temptation. Our job is to be alert and take advantage of His help! At first, you may not even recognize that God just helped you, and you may chalk it up to a "coincidence," but you will become more sensitive and observant as time goes on.

The ways of escape that God provides are very individualized and very creative, showing us a truly personal side of God. For example, if you have the stronghold of over-shopping and materialism, you may find yourself in a store, feeling the magnetic pull of the sale, and talking yourself into yet another unnecessary shopping spree. You pile your purchases on the counter and reach for your well-used debit card, only to remember that you loaned the card to one of your children that day. So you reach for a credit card, only to recall that you left it on the dresser that morning! Not to be discouraged, you pull out your phone to pay via an app, but your phone battery has died! As a last-ditch effort, you open up your wallet and discover that you only have a few dollars in cash. Finally, it dawns on you that maybe you should not be making this purchase, and you walk away from the store with the realization that God just provided you a way of escape from indulging in your stronghold!

Isn't it humbling and exciting to realize that God personally cares so much that He provides us a chance to escape from our temptation? Not just one chance, but even second, and sometimes third or fourth chances to tear our hearts away from our false idols? By obeying His ways of escape, you can now return home free from any guilt of overspending, and God might just open your eyes to discover that you already owned an article of clothing identical to what you were about to purchase!

In Jeremiah 17:9, the Bible tells us our hearts are deceitful above all things. Thru my experience, I have seen wholly devoted hearts...but I have also experienced semi-devoted hearts. I have observed selfish hearts, two-faced hearts, deceitful hearts, wishy-washy hearts, clogged hearts, and secretly ambitious hearts. For the most part, I do not believe we have a clue as to what our hearts are up to! Think about the past few weeks—it has been shocking to realize all the ways that our hearts have not been totally devoted to God.

In almost all of the cases of defective or disloyal hearts, the common denominator is that the person's undevoted heart has wandered to a horizontal relationship or devotion. It is called a lack of love for God. A horizontal devotion is a focus on what other people think, and a vertical devotion is a devotion to what God thinks. And take this further—if you allow your heart to be disloyal to God above, you will do it to others here on this Earth as well. For example, many couples make a lifelong, devoted commitment to one another before God, but then daily make a decision to side with the children at the expense of their spouse's feelings, or they allow their hearts to wander to a coworker at their

---

REMEMBER THAT FOR ALL STRONGHOLDS—NO MATTER WHAT THEY ARE—PURE FEELS BETTER THAN ANYTHING A STRONGHOLD CAN OFFER YOU!

---

job or to a neighbor down the street. These hearts have shifted from a vertical to a horizontal devotion, and it wreaks havoc. Romans 13:1 tells us that God has established all authorities here on this Earth, yet I have heard stories of employees becoming more devoted to one another than to the authorities God placed above them on the job, to the point of teaming up against a manager or company owner. It is a disloyal heart, a horizontal devotion versus vertical devotion.

Just as God designed our hearts to be devoted to *something* (that is why it is so easy to become addicted), God has designed our hearts to be able to be devoted to only *one thing*. The truth is, we have been trying for years to accomplish something that is simply an impossibility. It all boils down to the heart. The heart becomes divided because it is so easy to serve the one you love (your stronghold or idol), yet it is a problem to serve the Master you despise or reject. As long as you have a stronghold in your life, it will be an impossibility to stop serving the one you love…and it will be an impossibility to joyfully and competently serve the Master you despise. That is a characteristic of love.

You must realize this: you cannot "work" your way to Heaven. You cannot just go thru the motions and do the things you think God wants you to do, believing that will be enough love to show God. God is too smart to fall for that one. He can see right thru you if it is a chore to love Him with all your heart. Likewise, He can see when your obedience to Him is a work instead of a joy. If you love Him, you will obey Him, as it points out so clearly in John 14:15: *If you love me, you will obey what I command.* Stop working on the "have to" obedience and start working on the love…because when you choose to love God fully, the "want to" obedience just naturally follows! Fix the heart and your actions will follow.

Are you sick of what you have been doing? Then it is time to accept that you can completely be transformed by the renewing of your mind and focusing on God and Jesus Christ. I Peter 5:8-9 says *Be self-controlled and alert. Your enemy the devil prowls around like a roaring lion looking for someone to devour. Resist him, standing firm in the faith, because you know that your brothers throughout the world are undergoing the same kind of sufferings.* I Peter 4:7 says, *The end of all things is near. Therefore be clear minded and self-controlled so that you can pray.* You can do this! Just give your heart fully over to God, and then watch God change the inside of you by transforming your mind.

It helps to remember this—every time you pass a test or temptation, you will get a jewel straight from the Father! Some jewels are subtle; it could be just the peace of being in His will with no more guilt. Some jewels are extravagant, like large sums of money from an unexpected source or the restoration of a long-lost relationship. God has always rewarded me when I turn away from the things of this Earth and turn toward Him. I cannot emphasize this enough—I could fill up books with the rewards that He has given me. Remember when we talked about God's behavior modification? He created behavior modification, and He will reward your right choices! Open your eyes and recognize this extravagant and indulgent Heavenly Father who cannot wait to reward you when you abide in Him. *If you remain in me and my words remain in you, ask whatever you wish, and it will be given you,* Jesus tells us in John 15:7.

Jesus also explains in Matthew 7:9-11, *Which of you, if his son asks for bread, will give him a stone? Or if he asks for a fish, will give him a snake? If you, then, though you are evil, know how to give good gifts to your children, how much more will your Father in heaven give good gifts to those who ask Him!* God knows the best gifts, your favorite things, and how to indulge you with them. If you will just be patient and obedient, the jewels will blow you away! Keep your eyes open so you do not miss His sweet rewards—and His amazing ways of escape—and do not ever be afraid that God's results will disappoint your expectations. In fact, He will surprise you beyond your wildest dreams!

In summary, remember that for all strongholds—no matter what they are—pure feels better than anything a stronghold can offer you and better than grabbing greedily beyond God's boundaries. Eating just what the body needs feels better than overeating or starving yourself, spending an amount within your budget feels better than buying too much, obeying the sexual boundaries that God has given you within marriage (or even the boundary of abstinence if that is the case) feels better than sexual lust. Spending your time actively and productively feels better than squandering hours in front of your smartphone, computer screen, or gaming screen. Devoting yourself to building a family of peace, fun, and kindness feels *better* than nagging and control-ling and anger. When you overindulge in anything of the world, you are burdened with guilt and the lethargic feeling of never being able to break free—but when you turn away from idols and give your heart to God, you will be filled with unbelievable energy and no more guilt! The truth feels better than the lie, humility feels better than pride, and honest poverty feels better than dishonest gain. Just test it and see—God can do better than an alcoholic binge or an affair or a substance or social media, and He can provide everything you need for true happiness. Are you tired of trying to fill yourself up? Then unwind...surrender...give up and turn to God to fill your heart. Learn the joy of just letting God's approval and relationship be your everything in this desert of life. Drink from the only water in the desert—the living water that is Jesus Christ.

THOUGHT QUESTIONS

- What is the definition of denial that is given in this lesson?

  _____

  _____

  _____

  _____

- What are some ways that you have denied your own selfish desires this week?

  _____

  _____

  _____

  _____

  _____

- What was the result? Did you have any blessings from God related to your denial?

  _____

  _____

  _____

  _____

- Did you have some ways where you could have denied yourself and given to others, but you did not? What would you do differently next time?

  _____

  _____

  _____

- How did Christ deny himself for his friends and for all mankind?

  _____

  _____

  _____

  _____

  _____

- What are some areas where you still find yourself trying to play god, shift God's boundaries, or justify your selfish actions? What has been the result of those behaviors?

  _____

  _____

  _____

  _____

  _____

- Read 1 John 3:16-20. What does this scripture mean to you? Are there changes you can make so you can match the description in this scripture?

  _____

  _____

  _____

  _____

  _____

- Where have you been looking for excitement? Where are you looking for fulfillment and deep satisfaction? Do you think personal fulfillment comes in attaining a degree or striving for a leadership position at work? Is it in making it to the weekend so you can spend your time shopping or partying or binge-watching? What do you think about all day long? What great project is your goal in life?

_____

_____

_____

_____

- Whatever your pursuit—whether one the world considers admirable or not—do you feel deep satisfaction and contentment?

_____

_____

_____

_____

_____

- What are the true jewels of this life? Probably the way that I fell in love with God the most is by learning to recognize and appreciate His jewels that He gives me when I run toward Him and away from my false comforts or indulgences. God's personal "happies" or jewels are so individual and meaningful. You will recognize that it is God Himself giving you something, because only God knew how badly you wanted this particular "thing." God is rewarding you with your heart's desire for turning to Him. What are some of the rewards or jewels that you have experienced in the last few weeks from turning to Him instead of tasting and feeding off the world's pleasures?

_____

_____

_____

_____

- List all the ways of escape that God presented to you during this journey to help you break away from your stronghold. (For example: your stronghold might be overindulging in food, and one night as you were helping yourself to a double-serving of ice cream even though you were still full from dinner, your scoop of ice cream fell to the kitchen floor. Or, your stronghold might be alcohol, and you stopped by the bar for a so-called "well-deserved" drink, only to find the bar closed for a private party.) Did you recognize the way of escape and praise God for helping you turn away from your stronghold?

  _____

  _____

  _____

  _____

  _____

  _____

- If you feel like you gave in to your stronghold this week, list some of the ways you were not as successful as you had hoped. Write down what you think you could have done differently. What did you learn about yourself? Were there ways of escape that–looking back–you know God provided but you ignored at the time?

  _____

  _____

  _____

  _____

- Make a list of things you can do that will truly help you save your heart for the Father. (Some examples: If you feel the urge to open websites or apps you know you should not be looking at, delete those website links or apps and fill up your computer favorites or your app list with sites that are God-centered and will help you fill up on Him instead! If overusing alcohol or turning to recreational drugs in the evenings is your stronghold, remove those items from the house until you have more self-control. Pray for God to remind you to go for a walk every time you are tempted, and show God that you mean it by keeping your walking shoes and your earbuds right by the door!) Basically, you want to do everything you can to make choosing the stronghold more difficult and choosing God so much easier! God will reward every effort that you make to keep yourself battle-ready for all temptations.

_____
_____
_____
_____
_____
_____
_____

- Read Hebrews chapter 11 and describe the types of hearts that are portrayed in these great people of faith.

_____
_____
_____
_____
_____
_____

- Watch the reinforcement video "Save Your Heart for Me." According to the story of Chaucer and Virginia, what characteristic is a master looking for in a dog? In other words—if you have dogs of your own—why do you want them? Why do you crave their devotion? I will give you a hint—it is not because the dogs are so talented! Chaucer and Virginia would slobber all over everyone who came to visit, they stole the cats' food, and they barked at cars leaving the driveway instead of cars coming in. With all this in mind, what characteristic is a master really looking for in their pet?

_____

_____

_____

_____

_____

- Now for the parallel: What characteristic is God looking for in you? Does He want you for your musical talent or your academic achievement or your athletic coordination? I promise you, we humans are drooling and slobbering and nothing but trouble to the Father. So then, why is He waiting, looking out the window for us, like the father in the Parable of the Lost Son, waiting to bring our hearts home?[1] What defining characteristic is God looking for in us?

_____

_____

_____

_____

_____

_____

You can do this! You can give this to the Father! That is all He wants.

_____

1   *Luke 15:11-31*

- II Corinthians 10:5–6 says, *We demolish arguments and every pretension that sets itself up against the knowledge of God, and we take captive every thought to make it obedient to Christ. And we will be ready to punish every act of disobedience, once your obedience is complete.*
Write down your experiences, sharing every way that you were able to get your mind off your stronghold and place it on God and Christ. Take time also to share these experiences with your fellow program participants or on-line friends for encouragement!

"Take captive every thought" experiences:

_____

_____

_____

_____

_____

_____

_____

_____

_____

_____

- The verse in the last question paints a picture of an active, battle-ready soldier who is very prepared. Read Ephesians 6:10-18 describing the full armor of God. How does this passage describe being battle-ready for temptations and testing?

_____

_____

_____

_____

- A common lie that people often fight against is the lie that you are not worthy or special to God, but this simply is not true! If your heart were not a prize to be won, if you were not important to God, then why would satan want your devotion so badly? You are a prize to be won! Are there other lies in your mind that you find yourself listening to over and over? Record the lies below and write out the truths beside them. Whenever you hear a lie, quote the truth.

Lies: *(Example: I am not important to God; there is no way that I am special to Him.)*

_____

_____

_____

_____

_____

_____

_____

Truths: *(Example: I am a prize to God, so loved and special to Him! That is why this battle is so hard…God wants my devotion and I am being fought over!)*

_____

_____

_____

_____

_____

_____

_____

COUNTING YOUR BLESSINGS

Recognizing the countless blessings God has given you will be so important on this journey! Recount all the ways that God has blessed you, given to you, cared for you, and helped you. The more you fill in this list every day, the less magnetized you will be toward your stronghold. Spend extra time on your knees and on your face in prayer before the Father. Cry out to God and praise Him for letting you find Him and talk directly to Him. Think about it—it is so difficult to get close to famous people...yet here is the richest, most famous, most talented, and most well-known Being in the Universe, and He wants to hear from you, and He longs to have your love. Praise God for allowing you to get close to Him! Focus this week on the heavenly Father and Jesus Christ, and you will have a great week as you learn to approach each day, minute by minute, hour by hour!

_____

_____

_____

_____

_____

_____

_____

_____

_____

_____

_____

_____

COMMON STRUGGLE FOR LESSON 3

You have realized by now that you will have to make this Bible study and journey to the heart of the Father your top priority if you want to permanently break away from your strongholds. But if you are still struggling to get started by now, you have not taken this concept to heart. In the Parable of the Sower, found in Luke 8:4–15, Jesus talks about how easily the truth can be lost if it is not fully embraced. In the first and second soils, Jesus said seeds either did not sink in at all, or the seeds sprung up quickly in shallow soil, but because the message did not sink in, they withered away. This depicts the hearts that got excited about this relationship with God at first, but quickly gave in to struggles or gave up altogether when things got difficult. The third soil depicted the heart of someone who "gets it" and has been able to grow closer to the Father…but because this path was not their true priority, the things of the world eventually squeezed out and smothered the love for God. Like we mentioned before, you simply cannot love the world and God at the same time. You cannot have two masters like it says in Luke 16:13. If you are trying to keep your foot in both doors, I promise you that the love of the world will take over. Refocus, stand back up, and make the commitment to put God first above all else.

PRAYER

God, thank you for the blessing of saving your heart for me and not giving up on my heart yet. Dear Lord, please help me to make loving you my first priority. Please help me offer you the full devotion that you deserve. After all, you made me and created my heart to love, and you have spent countless hours caring for me and loving me, and you have even given your most prized possession—Jesus Christ—so that I can follow his example and keep my eyes adoringly fixed only on you. Thank you, God, for everything you have done in my life and especially for leading me on this journey. Thank you for the personal ways of escape you have provided and for the jewels that only you can give. Thank you for the blessing of salvation. I pray this in the name of Jesus Christ. Amen.

LESSON 4

FREEDOM OF THE MIND

SCRIPTURES

- [ ] Philippians 4:8-9
- [ ] Genesis 4:7
- [ ] Titus 1:15
- [ ] I Peter 2:9
- [ ] I Corinthians 6:12
- [ ] I Corinthians 10:23
- [ ] Ephesians 5:15-16
- [ ] II Timothy 2:22
- [ ] Psalm 119:37
- [ ] Psalm 90:12
- [ ] Psalm 127:2
- [ ] Proverbs 3:21–26
- [ ] Jeremiah 3:12-15

WEEKLY CHECKLIST

- [ ] Watch Lesson Four Video
- [ ] Answer Lesson Four Homework Questions
- [ ] Use your Reinforcement Resources

REINFORCEMENT RESOURCES

- [ ] *Weigh Down TV*—Watch "Teenage Role Models"
- [ ] *Weigh Down TV*—Watch Revolution Lesson 9, "Hyper Self-Focus"
- [ ] *Weigh Down Works!*—Read Chapter 15, "Love The Lord Your God With All Your Heart"

THOUGHTS FROM THIS LESSON

You have made it another week on this journey away from your strongholds! By now, you have hopefully discovered and experienced how personal God can be when you commit to putting Him first above all else! You are discovering how wonderful it feels to have more time, more energy, more peace—all because you gave up a stronghold that was pulling you down. Living a life fully devoted to God—heart, soul, mind, and strength—will be the most important calling you will have, and sadly, not many people today make this commitment.

We are called to be ambassadors of Christ and to represent God and His Kingdom, which puts us on a path of nobility. We can set ourselves firmly on this noble path, determined not to look to the right or the left at distractions, but unfortunately, living in today's society of social media and constant instantaneous interruption makes this challenge even more difficult. How can we fulfill this calling with so much instant public content, open for all the world to see? As for parents, what are your children being exposed to on social media, the internet, and video games?

For some of us, honestly, the pull of social media IS our stronghold. What is this drive for "likes" and "friends" and constant updates? With all this oversharing at our fingertips, it is highly possible that you are not only wasting your *own* time, but you could be intruding into God's time for other people when you interrupt their day to inform them of where you are going, what you are doing and what you are thinking. What are your posts actually pointing to? Do they only point back to you, and your material objects, and your own activities? What do your pictures tell people about you? Is your feed filled with selfies? Do your posts give your followers hope and encouragement, or did you waste their time or discourage them? Is that what you want to reflect with your life? What are you pointing people to…and why?

What about the impact of these posts on the next generation? Children are tech-savvy at younger and younger ages, and sooner or later they (and you) may be mortified when they see your posts, especially the posts you make about your children, including their embarrassing situations or revealing pictures of them, just to get "likes" for yourself.

Thanks to social media, what used to be saved in private, family baby books created for the child to see when they grow up is now out there for the world to see, to comment on, to mock. The scope and reach of the internet and social media is mind-boggling.

Video gaming has morphed into the same far-reaching anonymous community. What used to be individuals playing games in the living room has turned into real-time multiplayer connections of all ages and genders, a perfect anonymous platform. In addition, these multiplayer games create competition that leads to hours upon hours, even days upon days of gaming, all to impress an audience that is never actually seen, much like social media.

We and our children have never been so connected with the world, but what exactly are we getting into? How is this global social community affecting us and our children spiritually and emotionally? Our children are part of a unique generation—how does their maturity compare to the previous generations who were *not* addicted to photographs of themselves, constant comparisons, and anonymous platforms? Not only are children exposed to this community of "post anything, say anything," but they become potential victims for predators who use social media and gaming platforms to seek out their next target. We must wake up to what we are doing, where we are spending our time and focus, and what we are exposing our children to.

In addition to making this generation insensitive to time wasted scrolling from page to page, social media is also stretching the bounds of immodesty. It shows up in selfies, "likes," and the content you are scrolling. Only the Holy Spirit can give you the understanding of how wrong this lewdness is before God. Immodesty, lewdness, and coarse speech are almost unavoidable online and have become so much more socially acceptable. This is an abomination to the Kingdom of Good that God is trying to create. It is offensive, and it is tearing down God's House of beauty and nobility. Further, what adults do is mimicked by the children. Why are teenagers (and even younger children) so anxious to upload provocative pictures and expose themselves so much today? What is going on? And what is the future impact? Researchers are finding increasing negative effects on the mental health of our youth. The social media world of seeking instant acceptance impacts body image, expectations, sleep patterns, and mood—almost every area of their lives. Those addicted to social media fear they are being left behind, left out of activities or experiences–it is called the FOMO affect (fear of missing out). They worry they are missing or being left out, a fear of not being accepted or not being "good enough." Then they let satan's lies roll in, and instead of becoming proactive, they fall into the self-pity, victim mentality. This leads to posting more and more extreme updates or altered photos, trying to push themselves ahead, trying for more and more "likes."

When a person becomes self-focused and drawn into how many "likes" that they got on a post, this is a sideways-focus, a focus on praise of man and attention, a lust for recognition. Someone could be very self-assured and confident in terms of self-expression and self-identity, but somehow online, they forget all this, and they fall into the pull of the praise and recognition. Psychologists are continuing to point out the resulting anxiety, depression, self-identity conflicts, and body image issues. But what about the *spiritual* effect this has? What is happening to our hearts and the hearts of our precious children? Have parents underestimated the impact of vanity, the impact of crudeness? Are parents becoming numb to seriously shocking things that should remain private to that family?

Children are naturally at the age of learning; they are an open vessel, and there is incredible input available from God and His creation that they could be absorbing. Children *need* input, and as they say, a picture paints a thousand words. Curious children are learning about life, and so their curiosity draws them into interesting or fun photographs online, and then algorithms lead them into images and websites that may be on the edge…and then after that, with a touch of the finger, your child is being taken into a virtual world of the dark side—the worst images that you would never suspect would be out there, which then links to even more and more evil. It becomes a vacuum, stealing your kids away.

It is an insidious whirlpool that adults can get caught up in as well—phones and computers pulling them away from family life, lost in their apps and screens, texting, posting, gaming, fantasy sports, online shopping. This has resulted in a generation of spouses and children who feel neglected and lonely, even when their loved ones are right there in the room. This is a strong set-up for children who are desperate; they are starving for knowledge and acceptance and interaction, so they follow the example around them and start to explore the social world of the internet to fill in all the gaps. Without attentive parents there to connect with them and guide them to God to fill up their hearts and find their

---

THIS SOCIAL CONNECTION WITH GOD IS A WHOLE NEW PLANE...A WHOLE NEW PORTAL THAT ACTUALLY CAN COMMUNICATE STRAIGHT TO YOUR HEART AND HEAD.

---

true acceptance, this desire for interaction could make children seek attention from mankind over God. Then later, you will wonder why your child does not have a relationship with God or why they are disrespectful to their parents. Their absorbent minds have been filled with desires and lusts, with the need for approval from an anonymous audience, filled with bullying, anti-authority, and anti-parent concepts.

Too many parents today rely on these devices as babysitters, often occupying the children so they themselves can indulge time on their own devices. There is a strong connection between self-centered parents addicted to their screens and their children who get lost in a world of inappropriate interactions while they are right there in the same household, even at the same table. The internet is too dangerous at this point to be used as a babysitter! How wonderful it would be if once again a child's needs were fully met by attentive and loving parents, including the biggest need of all—this hunger, need, and desire to have a true and fulfilling relationship. It is one thing to be connected to an internet or a social media following, but you—as a God-focused parent—have a much better world to take them to, a right connection, an amazing instant feed, and that is the social media of God above. This social connection with God is a whole new plane, a whole new adventure, a whole new portal that actually can communicate straight to your heart and head, encouraging you and guiding you into good things. This connection does not come from a modem or a cable…it comes from the hovering, righteous parents, friends, and family members who are pointing the children and one another to a relationship with God above all other things.

Children learn to adore what their parents adore, so if you are seeing this behavior, this stronghold of the internet and social media, in your children, it is past time to look inward. If this is your stronghold, you must realize that feeling, that acceptance, that feedback you are looking for from your social media post or your game is never going to be found…there will be no end. That is why you keep reaching for the next level on the game or always thinking about creating your next post. Many who are caught up in gaming or constant social media attention end up loners, stuck in their rooms by themselves, stuck behind a false online persona. They equate "followers" as friends or "liking" a celebrity's post as real communication. They spend more time setting up a photo for their next post than they do interacting with the people around them. If this describes you, it is time to wake up. You could lose your spouse, your family, your friends, your job, your future opportunities and so much more if you do not wake up and change your direction, your mindset, and your heart. The good news is that it is not too late —you can do this today!

There is a Holy Spirit inside each person once they are born-again and living for God. Is that phone app, website, or social media page helping you or your children to be born-again? Is it supporting you or encouraging you on this journey to be more Christ-like? Instead of following people you do not even know online, you want to follow Christ, follow Paul, follow all the greats who lived their lives for God all these years! Follow the people around you today who are solid examples of obeying God and showing the fruits of the Spirit! They have focused on things much greater than what is on the latest news feed. Do you really think Christ or Paul or the Prophets would be caught up for hours with gaming or on social media? Would they have been over-shopping, overeating, overdrink-ing, or overdoing *anything*? No, they were on a pursuit to establish the Kingdom of the Most High God. Their instruction to us was: …*whatever is true, whatever is noble, whatever is right, whatever is pure, whatever is lovely, whatever is admirable—if anything is excellent or praiseworthy—think about such things. Philippians 4:8* They did not waste their minds nor their time on selfish indulgences because their mind and their time was not their own–they belonged to God. This is not your mind, and it is not your time. It is God's time, and it is God's mind.

Romans 12: 1-2 is very clear, *Therefore, I urge you, brothers, in view of God's mercy, to offer your bodies as living sacrifices, holy and pleasing to God—this is your spiritual act of worship. Do not conform any longer to the pattern of this world, but be transformed by the renewing of your mind. Then you will be able to test and approve what God's will is—his good, pleasing and perfect will.*

Set your mind on what is good, admirable, praiseworthy, and take your mind off the unnecessary, the garbage of the world. We need to be teaching our children right from wrong, how to think critically…but first we must master this ourselves. Teach your children these things, but also lead by example, because children are more apt to follow what you *do* rather than what you say. A heart trained up with the desire to be pure from within is the only hope. Just like you cannot take all the food or money or gossip that tempts you and lock it all away, the internet and social media is everywhere and it is here to stay. And it does fulfill many good and encouraging purposes when used correctly. To the pure all things are pure, and that is why being pure from within is the only hope I know.[1] Discover for yourself and then show your children that the internet and social media can be a portal to share good, wholesome, encouraging posts. Show them the Psalms, the Proverbs, what is good, what is bad, the difference in moral and immoral, learning how to deal with negativity, making sure they think thru all aspects of anything they post, and learning to refrain from cyber debates, cyber bullying, and cyber arguments. Your role as a parent is essential—monitoring time spent online, websites visited, the friends, the "likes," the "who" the child meets and interacts with online.

God wants us to love Him with all of our heart and our soul and our mind and our strength as we have read before, but how can anyone

---

1   *To the pure, all things are pure, but to those who are corrupted and do not believe, nothing is pure. In fact, both their minds and consciences are corrupted. Titus 1:15*

put this into practice if they are constantly running after what other people—even anonymous people—think of them? We should care more about what *God* thinks of us than any source on the internet. A royal priesthood is set apart and different from the world. What is a major difference between someone who is ignoble or corrupt versus a person who is Godly or noble? One heart is focused sideways, on other people and their false acceptance...but the other heart, the noble heart, is focused upward only, filled with encouragement, love, and worship for the One True God.

THOUGHT QUESTIONS

- What was your focus throughout this week? Where and how did you spend your time? What about the evening hours? Think back over the past few days and consider what you turned to when you had a few spare minutes (or maybe even when you needed to be doing other things)? Was it posting on social media, getting lost in other people's posts, scrolling thru apps, or picking up a gaming controller?

  _____

  _____

  _____

- If you have a screen time monitor, consider activating it and checking it at the end of each day or the end of the week to get a good picture of what you are really doing with your time. Make a log for when you open social media on your phone or spend personal time on your computer or other device. What does it tell you about your focus during your "free time"?

  _____

  _____

- Let's look again at II Corinthians 10. Write out verses 4-5 below.

  _____

  _____

  _____

- What does it mean to you to "take captive every thought"?

  _____

  _____

  _____

  _____

- Pray to God to show you what you could have been doing with that time that you spent on mindless scrolling or gaming or other distractions. Make a list here, and refer back to it anytime you find yourself drawn to distractions!

  _____

  _____

  _____

  _____

  _____

- Record some of the blessings that came from being more aware of how you spend your time and becoming more involved with your family, your home, your work, and your relationship with God.

  _____

  _____

  _____

  _____

- Read Isaiah chapters 30 and 31. According to these scriptures, what happens to people who depend upon and stay attached to Egypt (their stronghold)?

  _____

  _____

  _____

- As mentioned before, we all have to exist around our computers and our phones in this day and age. If you are having a hard time avoiding the app or the website or the game that has become your stronghold, try this! When you are on your device and that feeling or temptation comes over you, and you feel drawn strongly to go that direction, commit to fight thru it! Make note of the time and tell yourself you will not give in for the next 5 minutes! Ask God to show you how to devote that 5 minutes to actual work on your device, or to texting or calling a family member or friend who needs encouragement, to replying to a long overdue email, or to tackling a small housework chore. Then after 5 minutes, go another 5 minutes! (And remember to always look for those ways of escape that God provides...) The next thing you know, that original desire will fade away. Then the next time you feel that temptation, you will know how to fight this battle, and the desire will fade even more. Eventually, you will reach the point where you do not even know why you ever wanted to spend so much time on that game or that social media site!

  _____

  _____

  _____

  _____

  _____

COUNTING YOUR BLESSINGS

Recognizing the countless blessings God has given you will be so important on this journey! Recount all the ways that God has blessed you, given to you, cared for you, and helped you. The more you fill in this list every day, the less magnetized you will be toward your stronghold. Spend extra time on your knees and on your face in prayer before the Father. Cry out to God and praise Him for letting you find Him and talk directly to Him. Think about it—it is so difficult to get close to famous people...yet here is the richest, most famous, most talented, and most well-known Being in the Universe, and He wants to hear from you, and He longs to have your love. Praise God for allowing you to get close to Him! Focus this week on the heavenly Father and Jesus Christ, and you will have a great week as you learn to approach each day, minute by minute, hour by hour!

_____

_____

_____

_____

_____

_____

_____

_____

_____

_____

_____

_____

COMMON STRUGGLE FOR LESSON 4

The common struggle in this point of your journey is the desire to return to your stronghold for comfort. You may have gotten pretty good at resisting the temptation during the morning hours, maybe even thru the afternoon…but by 5 pm or so, you find your stronghold coming to mind more and more, calling your name. You find yourself battling the desire to overeat, binge-watch some mindless program, be rude to your family or spouse, show anger because something did not go your way, or lose yourself in websites or gaming. This is a strategic lesson. If you will stick with it, be steadfast, and prove your commitment to God even in the difficult hours, you will have made the right choice, and your heart will be uplifted!

You do not have to be perfect…there will be stumbles as you learn to redirect your heart. But when you finally catch on, the blessings will be so sweet that you will never want to look back. You have made some good changes and have seen some progress in the past weeks. Even tiny steps are to be celebrated! The only thing you could do wrong now is to give up or to quit—so hang in there! You can do this!

PRAYER

Dear Heavenly Father, help us all to hang in thru the temptations and the seemingly unrewarding times. Help us to see past the struggles to the victories. Help us to recognize even the smallest steps in the right direction, because it all helps us to appreciate the true life that comes from death to our selfish desires. We pray that we will never consider giving up this journey of turning our whole heart over to you. In Jesus' name, Amen.

LESSON 5

PURITY OF FOCUS

SCRIPTURES

- [ ] Colossians 3:5-10
- [ ] Deuteronomy 28
- [ ] Mark 7:20-22
- [ ] Galatians 5:19-21
- [ ] II Timothy 3:1-5
- [ ] Malachi 3:10
- [ ] Proverbs 6:15-19
- [ ] I Corinthians 6:12-18
- [ ] Proverbs 6:20-35
- [ ] Proverbs 7
- [ ] Job 31:1
- [ ] Luke 10:20
- [ ] Hebrews 13:4
- [ ] I Thessalonians 4:3-5
- [ ] Ephesians 5:1-10
- [ ] I Corinthians 7:2
- [ ] I Peter 2:11
- [ ] II Corinthians 12:21
- [ ] Revelations 22:15
- [ ] Ephesians 4:19

WEEKLY CHECKLIST

- [ ] Watch Lesson Five Video
- [ ] Answer Lesson Five Homework Questions
- [ ] Use your Reinforcement Resources

REINFORCEMENT RESOURCES

- [ ] *Weigh Down TV*—Listen to "How Can a Young Man Keep His Way Pure"
- [ ] *Weigh Down TV*—Listen to "Talks that Move Your Heart— Remove the High Places"
- [ ] *Rise Above*—Read Chapter 12, "Innocent in His Sight"

THOUGHTS FROM THIS LESSON

You have come so far on this journey away from your strongholds! Are you feeling more freedom, renewed peace, and even more joy as you have turned toward God? Are you experiencing blessings in ways you never even considered? In the same way, has it become more clear about the curses—the consequences—you had been experiencing when you had given your heart to your strongholds?

God has been showing you exactly what you have been giving your heart to over the past few weeks. You may have been very surprised at how much greed was exposed in your heart—greed for time, money, sex, food, substances, attention, control, etc. The New Testament describes greed as idolatry in Colossians 3:5: *Put to death, therefore, whatever belongs to your earthly nature: sexual immorality, impurity, lust, evil desires and greed, which is idolatry.* Why is greed considered idolatry? Greed is idolatry because we are grabbing things for ourselves rather than letting God provide exactly what we need. We are crossing His boundaries and taking things that are not ours to take. We are not depending upon our Creator to provide for us.

This tactic will never work, because we are only grabbing for false idols, and as we talked about earlier, false gods will never give back to you. False gods will never take away worldly desires, and in fact, just the opposite happens...you wind up only wanting more and more. To truly break away, you must set these idols aside and turn toward God, the only True God who can fill your heart to overflowing. Obedience to God includes a death to our own selfish will so that we can live for His will. And of course, to obey God means that we first need to know what He expects from us, what would please Him, and to find that out, we must stay in His Word!

God's Word is filled with descriptions of what can happen when we love Him fully and follow His will versus what can happen when we follow our own selfish will. The warnings from the prophets in God's Word were always about the blessings and the curses...blessings that we could expect when we obey God and His boundaries, and curses we could expect if we chose not to do that. Notice that the curses were always a longer list. Deuteronomy 28 is a great example of that—there are almost four times the warnings versus the beautiful persuasive words of reward. Why? It is because the warning was needed, and maybe it is needed even more in this generation than it was back in history. Those who have been living deep in sin do not believe that anything bad will ever really happen to them. If someone repeats a sin continually, the repetition of that sin does something to the mind. It makes the sin more comfortable and less dangerous. This is very scary, because eventually everything in God's Word will seem like mere idle threats that are never backed up. The consequences just will not seem real anymore until it is too late.

From the beginning of mankind, God has clearly listed the consequences of rebellion to Him and to His commands and boundaries. There are many lists of sins in God's Word, and the mention of sexual sins and lust always appears somewhere in each list, throughout the centuries of the Bible. Sexual sins are often spoken of more decisively and directly. *"Everything is permissible for me"—but not everything is beneficial. "Everything is permissible for me"—but I will not be mastered by anything. "Food for the stomach and the stomach for food"—but God will destroy them both. The body is not meant for sexual immorality...Flee from sexual immorality. All other sins a man commits are outside his body, but he who sins sexually sins against his own body. I Corinthians 6:12-13, 18*

There is no one with an excuse when it comes to sexual sins. The Bible has strong warnings against sexual desires that were outside of His boundaries. Even misplaced sexual desires that you do not act upon but entertain in your mind and heart are dangerous. In Matthew 5:27-28, Jesus states that entertaining lust in the heart toward someone is the same as adultery. *You have heard that it was said, "Do not commit adultery." But I tell you that anyone who looks at a woman lustfully has already committed adultery with her in his heart.* It is clear that this is something that was never intended in God's will.

Proverbs 6 and 7 reveal some of the characteristics of those caught up in sexual sins and make it clear that sexual sins must be handled swiftly and decisively. Repent and never ever dare to pick it back up again. You must commit yourself to keeping your actions, heart, and mind pure.

Again, Jesus said that the sin is in the heart—as we read above, even if you look at someone lustfully, you have sinned in the heart. There is hope, however! There is a way out. So what is the answer?

1. **Confess.** Confession means that you are ready to lay this sin down.

2. **Flee!** Get far away from whatever is causing you to click on that website, stop off at the adult bar, or gaze lustfully at a coworker. Get out of there. If this is happening in the office, it may be worth it to change jobs in order to save your marriage and your very soul. There must be urgent repentance, for this sin will destroy your very life, your salvation, your family and your livelihood. You could lose *everything*.

3. **Get wisdom.** Bind these scriptures to your heart. Write them down. Put them on your laptop and your phone. Set reminders to pop up throughout the day that bring up Proverbs 6 or other scriptures that will remind you to stay humble before God, that you are weak, that we are slow to learn. You fall in love with any stronghold by focusing on it and returning to it time and time again—in the same way, we need repetition, repetition, repetition of what God wants on our hearts and minds. Replace the lust with wisdom, and you will start to feel a new freedom, a new joy, and a new peace.

The pros and the cons—the rewards and the curses—are real and we are all left with an important choice in life. It is past time to stop and consider the outcome of your actions, to contemplate these serious consequences before you act. Stop yourself before you turn on that laptop or open that app. Stop it before you lust. Stop it before you enter into conversations that you should avoid. Stop yourself from getting into situations that flip on that lust. Just stop and take a different direction—do not let your feet rush into sin. Slow down. Stop. Then you will be forever changed. *Do not be deceived: God cannot be mocked. A man reaps what he sows. Galatians 6:7*

Sexual lusts can leave you feeling so guilty and can eat up your day, leaving you depressed and possibly even diseased. Stay away from that world. It is a sticky spiderweb, and once caught in it, the bites of injected poison of lies will bring the gentle, delicate souls closer and closer, poisoning them until they can no longer fight back. Open your eyes honestly, and you will see that you have spoiled yourself, you have grabbed for yourself more sexual pleasures than were perhaps allotted for one's lifetime (maybe even five lifetimes), just as the glutton has grabbed for themselves more food than they would need for two or even three lifetimes. Sexual greed does not satisfy; you will find yourself only wanting more and more and more. But today—if you reverse this process—you can find yourself wanting less and less, and you will feel the hope of freedom. When you do not put a log on the fire, the fire

YOU HAVE A SECOND CHANCE TODAY TO GET IT RIGHT—THIS VERY HOUR, THIS VERY MINUTE!

goes out. Stop adding fuel to this fire, and let God rebuild your heart and refill your soul so that you are not even tempted to look past what He has allotted for your life. People who push aside sexual lust—or any stronghold or greed—and pick up taking care of God's Kingdom are the ones who have been truly set free. Their focus is on God's will and His purpose all the time. They truly do not crave that lust anymore, for their eyes have been opened to how empty and dangerous it actually is.

When you live in God's will, He will provide everything you need, plus more. Look at His promise in Malachi 3:10: *'Test me in this,"* says the Lord Almighty, *"and see if I will not throw open the floodgates of heaven and pour out so much blessing that you will not have room enough for it."* That is amazing! Why want anything more than God's love and acceptance, to fly free from the sticky spiderweb world that wants to bring you down with it? You will find that when you first try to break away from your old life, your so-called "friends" may try to pull you back into the sin you shared. Do not fall for this! By being completely careful and finding friends who do not share in that sin, you can stay on the right path. Keep yourself away from the temptations and nearer to people who would not dare sin against God any longer.

Victory is possible for you, and you are so close! Do you know how many men and women have laid down sexual sins forever, never to pick them back up? We have beautiful testimonies of that success! God's people must be imitators of Him, as we are told in Ephesians 5:1-10: *Be imitators of God, therefore, as dearly loved children and live a life of love, just as Christ loved us and gave himself up for us as a fragrant offering and sacrifice to God.But among you there must not be even a hint of sexual immorality, or of any kind of impurity, or of greed, because these are improper for God's holy people. Nor should there be obscenity, foolish talk or coarse joking, which are out of place, but rather thanksgiving. For of this you can be sure: No immoral, impure or greedy person—such a man is an idolater—has any inheritance in the kingdom of Christ and of God. Let no one deceive you with empty words, for because of such things God's wrath comes on those who are disobedient. Therefore do not be partners with them. For you were once darkness, but now you are light in the Lord. Live as children of light (for the fruit of the light consists in all goodness, righteousness and truth) and find out what pleases the Lord.*

Praise God for His mercy, because if you are reading these words today, you have not died spiritually yet. You have a second chance today to get it right—this very hour, this very minute—and you have a chance to live a holy life for our God, for He deserves it!

THOUGHT QUESTIONS

- As you journey thru this desert, God will keep showing you exactly what you are giving your heart to. You may already be discovering things you had not realized about your heart before. What have you learned about where your heart is this week?

_____

_____

_____

_____

_____

- Read I Chronicles 28:9. Write it out below.

_____

_____

_____

_____

- Circle the action verbs above. What is this scripture calling you to do?

- In this lesson, we learned more about the warnings and the curses from sin. Read Deuteronomy 28 and list below some of the blessings and curses described in this passage:

Blessings:

_____

_____

_____

_____

_____

Curses:

_____

_____

_____

_____

• The consequences of sin are deadly, so we must put more energy into cleaning up our hearts and living pure lives. There are many lists of sins in the Bible that will help us realize how far-reaching this is. Read these passages and list out the sins they warn against:

☐ Mark 7:20-22   ☐ I John 2:16
☐ Galatians 5:19-21   ☐ Proverbs 6:16-19
☐ II Timothy 3:1-5   ☐ Matthew 15:19

_____

_____

_____

_____

• Read Proverbs 6 and 7. What are the characteristics and behaviors of someone caught up in sexual sin?

_____

_____

_____

_____

• One tip from this lesson was to keep encouraging and convicting scriptures in your heart by putting them where you will see them throughout the day—in your computer, on your phone reminders, etc. Read over the scriptures from this lesson and add them to your phone or computer to help you stay focused on this purity of the mind.

- If you seem to be constantly running back to your stronghold, remove yourself from that situation and spend your time encouraging or doing things for others. If you have time to devote to your strongholds, then you have time to do work for God's Kingdom instead! Honor the righteous, help the needy, and watch your tongue. James 1:26–27 says, *If anyone considers himself religious and yet does not keep a tight rein on his tongue, he deceives himself and his religion is worthless. Religion that God our Father accepts as pure and faultless is this: to look after orphans and widows in their distress and to keep oneself from being polluted by the world.* Watch your tongue, watch your thoughts, and watch how your time is spent.

- It helps to stay busy doing Kingdom work and serving others. What are some needs you can meet for your home, your family, your community, and God's Kingdom or positive things that you could be doing for others rather than indulging yourself?

_____

_____

_____

_____

_____

- Think about how often your mind wanders to your desires or your heart craves that stronghold you think is so well-hidden, and record the number of times each day you are having to battle temptation. Compare this to how you felt several weeks ago when you started this journey! The temptation should occur less and less—and will have a weaker pull each time—as the weeks go by. In a few more weeks, you can compare this number again and praise God for your progress.

- How often is your mind wandering to or craving your stronghold?

  _____

- How is this different from when you started?

  _____

  _____

  _____

- What changes are you making that have led to this difference?

  _____

  _____

  _____

  _____

- To help you go further, read the following passages:

  But you, brothers, are not in darkness so that this day should surprise you like a thief. You are all sons of the light and sons of the day. We do not belong to the night or to the darkness. So then, let us not be like others, who are asleep, but let us be alert and self-controlled. For those who sleep, sleep at night, and those who get drunk, get drunk at night. But since we belong to the day, let us be self-controlled, putting on faith and love as a breastplate, and the hope of salvation as a helmet. For God did not appoint us to suffer wrath but to receive salvation through our Lord Jesus Christ. I Thessalonians 5:4–9

  It is God's will that you should be sanctified: that you should avoid sexual immorality; that each of you should learn to control his own body in a way that is holy and honorable, not in passionate lust like the heathen, who do not know God; and that in this matter no one should wrong his brother or take advantage of him. The Lord will punish men for all such sins, as we have already told you and warned you. For God did not call us *to be impure, but to live a holy life. Therefore, he who rejects this instruction does not reject man but God, who gives you his Holy Spirit...Make it your ambition to lead a quiet life, to mind your own business and to work with your hands, just as we told you, so that your daily life may win the respect of outsiders and so that you will not be dependent on anybody. I Thessalonians 4:3–8, 11–12*

- After reading these passages, how much effort do you think we should put into the pursuit of a holy life?

  _____

  _____

  _____

  _____

- Read I Timothy 6:11-19. What does this passage tell you to pursue as part of this new life?

  _____

  _____

  _____

  _____

- As you continue to make these changes with your focus and your goals in life, these battles will soon be less intense, and as time passes, you will experience only occasional temptations that do not have the intensity of your current battles. The fire will die out if you do not fan the flame. Make sure you are clearing your mental schedule for this journey, for nothing is more important than learning to love God with all of your heart, all of your mind, all of your soul, and all of your strength.

COUNTING YOUR BLESSINGS

Recognizing the countless blessings God has given you will be so important on this journey! Recount all the ways that God has blessed you, given to you, cared for you, and helped you. The more you fill in this list every day, the less magnetized you will be toward your stronghold. Spend extra time on your knees and on your face in prayer before the Father. Cry out to God and praise Him for letting you find Him and talk directly to Him. Think about it—it is so difficult to get close to famous people...yet here is the richest, most famous, most talented, and most well-known Being in the Universe, and He wants to hear from you, and He longs to have your love. Praise God for allowing you to get close to Him! Focus this week on the heavenly Father and Jesus Christ, and you will have a great week as you learn to approach each day, minute by minute, hour by hour!

_____

_____

_____

_____

_____

_____

_____

_____

_____

_____

_____

COMMON STRUGGLE FOR LESSON 5

If you find you have not made many positive changes or are still struggling this far into the Strongholds program, the most common obstacle is an overwhelming desire within your heart to blame someone or something else for the fact that you are still slandering, cursing, vaping, focused on money, overindulging in food or alcohol, controlling your family with anger, or being given over to sexual sins or other stronghold. You want to blame anyone or anything other than yourself. This is called "projection," and it is often accompanied by a deep-seated, bubbling cauldron of anger. This anger will surface unexpectedly from time to time when you struggle with trying to lay down the idols you still love. You will feel mad at this program, mad at me, mad at other participants who are doing well, mad at your spouse when they ask how the lessons are going, mad at other people who are not controlled by your stronghold...and you will even feel mad at God.

My friends, stop blaming everyone else. Please take this energy and get mad at your own stronghold! Get mad at this false comfort, false god, and false lover. This anger—when properly focused on the right thing, your sin—will help you turn away from secretly running to your stronghold and instead turn your love and attention toward God. A rush of joy will fill your heart when you do this, because God will not let that heart-change and behavior go without great reward.

PRAYER

Dear God, please help us focus our eyes and hearts off the things and the people of this world, and help us focus only on you. Help us to focus on just your adoring eyes and your will for us, and help us to repent from our selfish attitudes and behaviors. Help us to walk out in faith this week so we can experience the great reward that you have promised when we turn to you. Help us to be honest with ourselves and to project any anger where it truly needs to be, toward anything that is separating us from your Love. Amen.

POSITIVE HEART AND BEHAVIOR CHANGE LIST

Write down your positive heart and behavioral changes. Some changes will be emotional or mental, some will be spiritual, and some will be related to your physical and spiritual strength. Think and write, then think and write some more! Let God open your eyes to the ways this stronghold is affecting you and the people around you.

_____

_____

_____

_____

_____

_____

_____

_____

_____

_____

_____

_____

_____

_____

_____

_____

_____

_____

_____

_____

LESSON 6

A JOYFUL SPIRIT

SCRIPTURES

- [ ] Genesis 4:2-16
- [ ] Psalm 42:11
- [ ] Revelation 21:4
- [ ] Isaiah 26:3
- [ ] Psalm 34:17
- [ ] Galatians 5:22-23
- [ ] John 15:11
- [ ] Hebrews 12:2

- [ ] Romans 14:17
- [ ] Psalm 126:2
- [ ] John 16:33
- [ ] Deuteronomy 30:1-10
- [ ] Jeremiah 6:16
- [ ] Proverbs 3:21-26
- [ ] Isaiah 66:2

WEEKLY CHECKLIST

- [ ] Watch Lesson Six Video
- [ ] Answer Lesson Six Homework Questions
- [ ] Use your Reinforcement Resources

REINFORCEMENT RESOURCES

- [ ] *Weigh Down TV*—Listen to "Self-focus, Self-Pity and Depression"
- [ ] *Weigh Down TV*—Watch *History of the One True God*, Lesson Five: "The Cain Test"
- [ ] *Weigh Down TV*—Watch "How to Overcome Depression and Anxiety"
- [ ] *Weigh Down Works!*—Read Chapter 19, "Free From Unwanted Behaviors and Substances"

THOUGHTS FROM THIS LESSON

When you first began this *Freedom From Strongholds* Series, you started soaring above the temptations, filled with hope and joy! Then you hit that hot Desert of Testing, and you experienced just how strongly your idols are holding on to your heart and mind. By now, you may be wondering if you are getting anywhere with these lessons. But never lose hope! Just realizing the *truth* is your first step to freedom. Staying honest and not blaming others is important. However, this is not a program where you have an exam or some outward measurement to let you know how much you have changed. This is a *heart* program, and you measure success by the *fruit* in your life—which includes love, joy, peace, patience, kindness, goodness, faithfulness, gentleness and self-control.[1] Even if you have just felt more peace and love since starting this Series, then you are going in the right direction!

The Bible teaches us that moderation is the key. "Moderation" may be a gray term in the beginning, especially in the areas of things we must do every day. Where is "too much" spending, "too much" food to eat, "too much" talking, etc.? Where are the boundaries in this freedom in Christ? The boundaries are the boundaries of *love*—and you know when your heart is turning toward God, and you know when your heart is not. You can feel it inside as your stronghold has less power over you; you can feel God's Spirit guiding you more and more!

There are some people taking this class who suspect deep down that their heart for their stronghold has not changed at all. The fact is, the road out of this prison of your stronghold can have many side streets that beckon you or distract you from leaving. If you continue to hold on to any bit of your stronghold—your overspending, overdrinking, eating disorder, smoking/vaping, seeking the praise of other people, gossip, anger, gambling, sexual sins, gaming, etc.—you will find yourself pulled into some dangerous side streets called sin, guilt, depression, and anger. Until you feel true repentance in your heart, you will remain stuck at these crossroads, and it is a painful place to be...afraid to turn back but

---

1   *See Galatians 5:22-23.*

afraid to fully give up your past idols. What if God does not take care of you? What if you do not feel the love everyone else is feeling? What if you just cannot do it?

The key to unlocking many of these prison doors is found in one of my favorite scriptures, 1 John 4:16–18: *God is love. Whoever lives in love lives in God, and God in him. In this way, love is made complete among us so that we will have confidence on the day of judgment, because in this world we are like him. There is no fear in love. But perfect love drives out fear, because fear has to do with punishment. The one who fears is not made perfect in love.*

So perfect love—or wholehearted love—drives out fear. I challenge anyone who feels trapped to spend some time getting to know God so you can experience this true give-and-take relationship. A whole heart of love for the Father gets rid of all fear, because you have faith that He will take care of you. The things of the world will call you back and confuse you, but you must listen to the right voice, the voice of God's Spirit, that is trying to keep you on the right path. Proverbs 3 assures us by saying, *My son, preserve sound judgment and discernment, do not let them out of your sight; they will be life for you, an ornament to grace your neck. Then you will go on your way in safety, and your foot will not stumble; when you lie down, you will not be afraid; when you lie down, your sleep will be sweet. Have no fear of sudden disaster or of the ruin that overtakes the wicked, for the Lord will be your confidence and will keep your foot from being snared. Proverbs 3:21–26*

The answer is the same for all who struggle—every prisoner needs to seek out and set forth on the narrow path that leads to God. It all boils down to the fact that we are looking for a feeling of acceptance. It is a warm, loving feeling high up in our heart. Guilt is an ugly feeling, and we may be trying all the wrong methods to get rid of it. As we continually choose our own desire over God's will, it just leads to more and more guilt and depression. Ultimately, after we have continually looked for every excuse, we must face the fact that we simply do not want to give up our idols.

In the past lessons, we have talked specifically about Deuteronomy 28 (as well as many other passages), where the Bible tells us clearly that we will experience painful consequences for our sins. We have all felt this pain that comes from following our own selfish choices, and we have all turned to worldly solutions to alleviate or fill that pain, but the answer is not going to be found in the world. In fact, the world is only going to offer you a solution that will ultimately make you worse...and that is an even *deeper* focus on yourself and your own problems: the "take care of yourself, put yourself first" mentality. This solution only leads you down another dangerous side street, carrying you further away from God.

Covering up your feelings of guilt with projection, dishonesty, drugs, self-pity, and other strongholds are not the treatments I recommend. However, turning a whole heart to God can bring a rush of joy, filling up the areas where guilt and depression were once dominant. In its place will be a heart filled with unspeakable happiness and contentment! There will always be a one-to-one ratio between joy and full obedience to God—a heart that yields to the Father in love and true repentance will always be fulfilled and peaceful.

Years ago, I turned from the stronghold of overeating (which boils down to greed for more food than my body needed), and God filled

---

GOD WANTS TO BE YOUR EVERYTHING. HE WANTS TO FULFILL YOUR DESIRES AND DREAMS.

---

up each and every day so efficiently that I never felt tempted to turn back to food as a stronghold! I discovered very quickly that God could do so much better than the extra food ever could, and I experienced freedom from the guilty feelings and true joy at being free from that stronghold. Over the decades, I have found that seminar participants who have been able to turn *permanently* from their stronghold are those who genuinely believe that what God has asked them to do is better, superior, more peaceful, and more fun than any stronghold they had been holding on to. What words do I have to use to convince you? Why don't you just try it? Keep in mind that you may not experience all these emotions in the first 15 minutes after you repent and turn and apply God's ways...oh, no! This will be a test, and you may have to wait for a while, because God wants to see if you are truly serious this time about laying down your stronghold for good. But those who wait on the Lord will be rewarded—that is His promise. *He gives strength to the weary and increases the power of the weak. Even youths grow tired and weary, and young men stumble and fall; but those who hope in the Lord will renew their strength. They will soar on wings like eagles; they will run and not grow weary, they will walk and not be faint. Isaiah 40:29-31*

What we have learned about God is that He wants to be your everything; He wants to fulfill your desires and dreams. Do you want to take a walk? He wants to go with you. Do you have a good joke? He wants to be in on it. Do you have a difficult task at work? He wants to help you thru it! Are you bored? He wants to help you fill your time! He can fix anything, He can find anything, and He wants to get you to a point where He is your first thought in every occasion…not just somewhere to turn as a last resort.

True repentance from your sins is a commitment—it means you are making the choice to *never* do it again. True repentance means returning to God fully, so building this relationship with Him will require letting go of your own selfish wants and desires, giving up your own will, and seeking out and doing God's Will. "Giving up your own will" sums up how Christ lived on this Earth. In Luke 22:42, Christ was aware that His next step was crucifixion, but He prayed, *Father, if you are willing, take this cup from me; yet not my will, but yours be done.* And in John 6:38, Jesus said, *For I have come down from heaven not to do my will but to do the will of him who sent me.* Over and over and over, Jesus talked about giving up his will and doing the Father's will. Giving up our will is repenting; it is turning and doing things God's way. This can sound easy…until that moment comes when God's will and your will do not match up. That is the testing moment where God is waiting to see what direction you will choose.

This lesson—and in fact, this whole Strongholds Series—is all about crying out to God, for He will be the only Deliverer. *The righteous cry out, and the Lord hears them; he delivers them from all their troubles. Psalm 34:17* No stronghold will save you from your troubles, because only God has all the answers, and He has been here for all time. You cannot find the answers thru feeling sorry for yourself or worried about yourself, or by projecting blame onto other people, or by feeling angry or depressed. God is trying so hard to pull you out of yourself and bring you to Him. You are valuable to Him, and He has been giving you ways of escape and rewards for even the smallest acts of obedience to His boundaries! Look around, and worry more about God and others than you do about yourself...and the next thing you know, you are walking on the right path to being completely set free.

For my yoke is easy and my burden is light. Matthew 11:30 Take on the yoke of Jesus Christ, because the result in turning to God is going to be the joyful fruits of the Spirit. The one true path for joy, contentment, peace, and love is following the heart of Jesus Christ—all the way to the heart of the Father.

THOUGHT QUESTIONS

- Read the story of Cain and Abel in Genesis 4 to see how Cain was not obeying God wholeheartedly. His brother, Abel, pleased God by bringing Him the best of the best for an offering, while Cain only brought what he himself wanted to offer God. Cain became angry with his brother who offered God the best he had. Write down the response of Cain and what you have learned about his motivations.

  _____

  _____

  _____

- Have you felt like Cain in the past? Have you felt jealousy or anger toward others who are doing things right and being blessed for it?

  _____

  _____

  _____

- God told Cain, *"Why are you angry? Why is your face downcast? If you do what is right, will you not be accepted? But if you do not do what is right, sin is crouching at your door; it desires to have you, but you must master it."* What do you think this means? What was God telling Cain to do?

_____

_____

_____

_____

• Do you ever feel that God has not accepted you? Do you feel at arm's length from God? Do you feel as if you simply are not as devoted or as excited about God as some of your other Christian friends? Try to express what your own personal relationship with God is, then ask God to help you figure out what could be keeping you from being the true apple of His eye.

_____

_____

_____

_____

_____

• I discovered that when I obeyed God's Word and followed His Spirit, I grew closer to Him. Obedience and love walk hand-in-hand. Read the following passages on obedience to God to see how connected it is to the love relationship you are developing with Him. Remember that when you love Him, you will obey Him. Keep working on the love for God, and your passion for the stronghold will disappear.

II Chronicles 31:21: In everything that he undertook in the service of God's temple and in obedience to the law and the commands, he sought his God and worked wholeheartedly. And so he prospered.

Romans 6:16: Don't you know that when you offer yourselves to someone to obey him as slaves, you are slaves to the one whom you obey—whether you are slaves to sin, which leads to death, or to obedience, which leads to righteousness?

John 14:15: If you love me, you will obey what I command.

John 15:10: If you obey my commands, you will remain in my love, just as I have obeyed my Father's commands and remain in his love.

- In Matthew 9:12-13, Jesus said: "*It is not the healthy who need a doctor but the sick. But go and learn what this means: 'I desire mercy, not sacrifice'. For I have not come to call the righteous, but sinners.*" God does not care if you are rich or poor, famous or unknown, etc. He only cares about your heart. Read Psalm 139 and write down how you see yourself in God's eyes now.

  _____

  _____

  _____

  _____

- True repentance is misunderstood; otherwise, we would have seen more of it by now! II Corinthians 7:8–11 says: *Even if I caused you sorrow by my letter, I do not regret it. ...I am happy, not because you were made sorry, but because your sorrow led you to repentance. For you became sorrowful as God intended and so were not harmed in any way by us. Godly sorrow brings repentance that leads to salvation and leaves no regret, but worldly sorrow brings death. See what this godly sorrow has produced in you: what earnestness, what eagerness to clear your-selves, what indignation, what alarm, what longing, what concern, what readiness to see justice done. At every point you have proved yourselves to be innocent in this matter.*

- This passage describes two types of sorrow: "Godly sorrow" and "worldly sorrow." When you have Godly sorrow, it leads to permanent change. What is the difference between the two?

  _____

  _____

  _____

  _____

- Examine your heart to determine honestly if you have been truly sorry before the Father. Read the following scriptures and notice how these individuals immediately repented and turned to God when their sin was exposed before Him. Use the space provided to comment on these examples.

  Luke 3:1–18:

  _____

  _____

  John 8:1–11:

  _____

  _____

  Luke 19:1–9:

  _____

  _____

  John 4:6–26:

  _____

  _____

Acts 2:37–41:

_____

_____

- Read Psalm 78 and describe the pattern of behavior exhibited by the children of God:

_____

_____

_____

- List the concepts from Psalm 78 that will help you avoid repeating the actions of the Israelites.

_____

_____

_____

_____

- What are some situations that have caused you to feel self-pity, anxiety or depressed in your own life?

_____

_____

_____

_____

- How can you prepare to respond differently to those same tests going forward?

_____

_____

_____

COUNTING YOUR BLESSINGS

Recognizing the countless blessings God has given you will be so important on this journey! Recount all the ways that God has blessed you, given to you, cared for you, and helped you. The more you fill in this list every day, the less magnetized you will be toward your stronghold. Spend extra time on your knees and on your face in prayer before the Father. Cry out to God and praise Him for letting you find Him and talk directly to Him. Think about it—it is so difficult to get close to famous people...yet here is the richest, most famous, most talented, and most well-known Being in the Universe, and He wants to hear from you, and He longs to have your love. Praise God for allowing you to get close to Him! Focus this week on the heavenly Father and Jesus Christ, and you will have a great week as you learn to approach each day, minute by minute, hour by hour!

_____

_____

_____

_____

_____

_____

_____

_____

_____

_____

_____

COMMON STRUGGLE FOR LESSON 6

Many times by this point in the Series, if we have been doing well, we start to become overly confident in being able to overcome our stronghold. We say to ourselves, "Hey, I get this concept. I can tackle this problem any time I get ready," and then we relax. We let our guard down. We let ourselves have little cheat-days here and there, we loosen our resolve a bit more. Then we tell ourselves, "I will just start over on Monday!" When we say we are going to "start over on Monday," what we are really saying is that we are not going to do it because we do not want to do it. If we *did* truly want to get it right, we would change now, this very minute! We do not realize that we are merely lying to ourselves. But we must never forget that satan is the father of lies as it says in John 8:44, and satan would love for us to become overly secure and self-assured to the point that we ease up in breaking away from our stronghold. Please do not play around, become too relaxed, or flirt too much with the world, and never become too sure that you can just cheat sometimes and break away whenever you want to. Our hearts are tricky things. Jeremiah 17:9 says, *The heart is deceitful above all things and beyond cure. Who can understand it?*

PRAYER

Dear God, please help us to realize how conniving, deceptive, and dishonest our own hearts can be when we are still holding on to our stronghold, and help us to realize that satan is constantly lying to us. Help us to take our entire heart, soul, mind, and strength and turn it all toward you, not toward ourselves or toward things of this world. Guide us to make it past the crossroads and sidestreets that want to pull us onto dangerous pathways and distract us from our true purpose. Help us take the time to be still so that we may hear your voice of truth thru your creation and thru your Word. Jesus, you are the Way, and the Truth, and the Life. Help us depend upon and focus on you and your example at all times. Amen.

A LIFE OF PEACE

SCRIPTURES

- ☐ Matthew 5:21-22
- ☐ Romans 12:1-21
- ☐ Psalm 4:4
- ☐ Psalm 37:8
- ☐ Proverbs 15:1
- ☐ Proverbs 19:11
- ☐ Proverbs 22:24
- ☐ Proverbs 29:8, 11
- ☐ Ecclesiastes 7:9
- ☐ James 1:19-20
- ☐ James 4:1-2
- ☐ Psalm 86:15
- ☐ Psalm 103:8
- ☐ Proverbs 16:32
- ☐ I Peter 2:23
- ☐ I Corinthians 13:4-7
- ☐ Ephesians 4:31-32
- ☐ Colossians 3:8
- ☐ I Timothy 2:8

WEEKLY CHECKLIST

- ☐ Watch Lesson Seven Video
- ☐ Answer Lesson Seven Homework Questions
- ☐ Use your Reinforcement Resources

REINFORCEMENT RESOURCES

- ☐ *Weigh Down TV*—Listen to "A Life of Anger and Rage Vs. a Life of Gentleness"
- ☐ *Weigh Down TV*—Listen to "Love your Neighbor as Yourself"
- ☐ *Weigh Down TV*—Watch *Life with Gwen and Joe,* "The Importance of Christ-like Words and Speech"
- ☐ *History of the Love of God*—Read Chapter 18, "The White Light of Christ"

THOUGHTS FROM THIS LESSON

Refrain from anger and turn from wrath. Do not fret – it leads only to evil. Psalm 37:8

The world is growing angrier every day. We see it around us everywhere we turn…at the workplace, in the community, on our roads, across the internet, and increasingly, right in our own homes. Viral videos of customers and employees berating each other are circulating globally; employers and employees face wrath every day on the job as workplace rage resulting in violence is skyrocketing. Road rage stories are sadly commonplace as tempers rise on our streets and highways. Internet haters and bullies seem to have free reign in their anonymous posts and comments. We have all experienced being wronged or treated unfairly at some point in life, but must be on guard, for our own private rages, furious resentments, or building jealousies can foster hatred in our own hearts, and as the Bible teaches us, that is the same as murder: *Anyone who hates his brother is a murderer, and you know that no murderer has eternal life in him. I John 3:15* Human nature wants to return anger with anger, but even in Jesus' first sermon, he warns that this anger could jeopardize our eternal life: *I tell you that anyone who is angry with his brother will be subject to judgment. Again, anyone who says to his brother, "Raca," is answerable to the Sanhedrin. But anyone who says, "You fool!" will be in danger of the fire of hell. Matthew 5:22*

Despite these Biblical warnings, many people justify their anger and cannot seem to let it go. These inner feelings of justification and desire for revenge that result from anger usually mean that the world centers around you and the belief that you "deserve" something. It is largely projection—you do not know how to handle the feelings of not getting what you feel you deserve, so you compensate by pushing anger and blame outward toward others. You live with a readiness to attribute anything that happens to you as someone else's fault, which means that anyone around you could be at fault at any time. *They* are the problem and the cause of your misfortunes.

The only way to turn this whole thing around is to look inward and start over. Slow down. Learn to recognize this feeling when it rises up in your heart, and then once it is identified, you have to flip your perspective. You are essentially starting your whole life over, because life will no longer be about you. Start telling yourself, "I am here to make *God* look good." It is not our job to savor the self-focused feeling of taking our anger out on someone else. It is not our right or our purpose in life to do this. Ask yourself, "Who am I, that I would take out my anger or disappointment on another human being made by God?"

Maybe you are not mistaken that you have been treated wrongly or that someone else needs to be corrected, but think about this Scripture: *...first take the plank out of your own eye, and then you will see clearly to remove the speck from your brother's eye. Matthew 7:5b* Ninety-nine percent of the time, there is a log in our own eye, with only the speck in another's. That log of "self" must go. Just start over and every time you think about yourself or how you have been wronged in some way, stop. Stop right there and instead think about God...how does He feel? How is He going to look? Are you ruining His whole project? He made the Earth. These are His battles, and He is the General. This entire world is a battle of satan against God. Yes, satan does swoop in against the Saints whom God created, but the overall war is God's! We should look to Christ, the firstborn over all Creation, as our example. When people persecuted him, even he did not consider himself someone with a right to retaliate. *Instead, he entrusted himself to him who judges justly. I Peter 2:23* Christ turned the other cheek and trusted in God for judgment upon those who mistreated him. He never sought revenge.

As we have discussed before, we need to take every thought captive, as we are taught in II Corinthians 10:5, and then make sure that we are seeing the situation from God's perspective. There is a purpose behind everything God allows. If someone cuts in front of you on the road, maybe that saved you from a speeding ticket or an accident. Something that "gets in our way" could have been an angel. Slowing down is one of the biggest things that we all need to do, so anything put in our path to slow us down is beautiful and should never cause us to feel angry. The angels are around you. Everything has a spiritual purpose.

You are here for God, and that is why you can be so happy every day because every day you are not living for what you "think" you deserve, but you are living to make God look good. Those old feelings of anger and rage will dissipate, and your shame and anxiousness will disappear, soon to be only a distant memory. God is there quickly to turn it all around for those who are looking to Him.

Just as with the other strongholds we have discussed in this Series, letting go of anger, judgmentalness, and self-focus comes down to a choice, and the amazing twelfth chapter of Romans teaches us how to make this choice and what to do with all the emotions we have inside of us. It starts with, *Therefore, I urge you, brothers, in view of God's mercy…* So before we can go any further, we must begin by recognizing the wondrous mercy of God. Start by imagining yourself as the chiefest of sinners. What if you had murdered people, hurt others, been cruel or abusive or stolen from someone. Imagine if you then find out you have a chance at redemption—you have one shot at getting all your crimes and your sins completely wiped clean, a blank slate, and with your reputation cleared? Your record would be spotless again. You would have the chance to accept this mercy and totally transform your life with a chance to live forever! How would you respond? I cannot understand why we all do not fall down on our faces daily in appreciation and praise, and then do everything that we possibly can to live a completely transformed life, so appreciative of this one shot we have been given. We should all be making our very best effort to get every word, every thought, and every action completely right before God, because we want this chance to live forever.

Paul is pleading with us as he continues, *Therefore, I urge you, brothers, in view of God's mercy, to offer your bodies as living sacrifices, holy and pleasing to God… Romans 12:1a* We are to offer our entire bodies– heart, mind, and strength, from our head to our feet–in everything that we are doing, during all our hours in the day and all our days in the week. We are to throw everything into this effort to live for God…dropping everything that distracts us from this purpose. Throw everything into your new life as a living sacrifice for God.

Paul continues that thought with ...*this is your spiritual act of worship. Do not conform any longer to the pattern of this world but be transformed by the renewing of your mind.* Romans 12:1b-2a "The renewing of your mind"—that is what you are doing right now in this Series! Your life is being transformed by what you are learning, and you are not going to conform to the pattern of the world any more. In other words, drop that old focus! Get out of it. Forget the world. Let it go. It is time to change and move on. Do not let the world shape your thoughts, your mind, or your actions any longer. This might sound impossible and you might have tried in the past but failed, but did you truly *renew your mind* in those past efforts? Take this chance and tell yourself, "I am going to do it right for God this time. I am going to love Him with all my heart. I am not going to mess up anymore. I am going for it. I am going to transform!" When you do not conform to the world anymore and

DO NOT BE DOWNCAST OR DISCOURAGED BY THE WORLD. DO NOT LET EVIL OVERCOME YOU. JUST FIND A WAY TO DO GOOD TODAY.

you commit to getting everything right, guess what happens? *Then you will be able to test and approve what God's will is—his good, pleasing and perfect will.* Romans 12:2b You will begin to feel God's Spirit in you, you will know the path He wants you to take in every situation, and you will experience that amazing feeling of walking in the will of the Father!

As we mentioned above, the fact is that sometimes you will experience being treated unfairly or unkindly by someone else. In the past, you would have allowed anger to flare up and you would project outward. But now, let's look back to Romans 12 for direction on how to interact with those around us, especially when we have been treated unkindly: *Bless those who persecute you; bless and do not curse. Rejoice with those who rejoice; mourn with those who mourn. Live in harmony with one another. Do not be proud, but be willing to associate with people of low position. Do not be conceited. Do not repay anyone evil for evil. Be careful to do what is right in the eyes of everybody. If it is possible, as far as it depends on you, live at peace with everyone. Do not take revenge, my friends, but leave room for God's wrath, for it is written: "It is mine to avenge; I will repay," says the Lord. On the contrary: "If your enemy is hungry, feed him; if he is thirsty, give him something to drink. In doing this, you will heap burning coals on his head." Do not be overcome by evil, but overcome evil with good. Romans 12:9-21*

When we are mistreated or wronged, our worldly flesh wants to get revenge or vindication. In our society, we can turn to the justice system to seek legal protection, amends, or justification when we have been misused or harmed. It seems in today's world, however, we are experiencing a broadening level of injustice, and sometimes it seems we cannot count on the courts to uphold righteousness. This is nothing new, as there are many Biblical scriptures related to how it often appears that those who are evil or greedy seem to prevail in this earthly world. The wonderful news is that there is a Higher Court and there is always true justice in that Court! God sits on His Throne in the courtroom of the Kingdom of Love, and He is very clear about what is going to happen for those who love Him with a committed heart…and what is in store for those who do not.

We cannot overcome evil with evil. In fact, that is what the world does, and we are not going that direction anymore. As Paul wrote, we are to overcome evil with good. We are to repay the actions of our enemies with kindness, and then look at what happens: *In doing this, you will heap burning coals on his head.* So it is the opposite of what you think! They are not getting away with anything. Look at what your kindness is doing. You just keep giving, turning the other cheek, and keep praying for those who persecute you, and allow God to do His work.

Keep in mind that Paul also tells us not to be proud or conceited. The truth is that if you really think back and contemplate everything you have either done or have desired to do in the past, you should be so humbled. We all know we have done wrong, we have acted rashly, we have treated others unfairly, we have done shameful things in anger or wrongful judgment, and we need mercy. Again, look at the first line in

Romans 12:1 again: *in view of God's mercy.* We have been shown so much mercy from God, and we are to extend that mercy to those around us.

Oh, if we could just throw everything down! Get rid of the world and start a new life. Get it all right in our heart and our actions. We have an opportunity to do just that! Let's go for it and run this race of life like we are running for the gold, not for second or third place. Pick yourself up! Get into the race, and go for it. Do not be downcast or discouraged by the world. Do not let evil overcome you. Just find a way to do good today. Bless those who persecute you. Pray for others and pray for God's Spirit to guide you. Look for God's ways of escape when you are tempted. Do not let anger, jealousy, judgmentalness, or self-focus overcome you today. Just do what is right!

We can do this. This mindset and life for God unites us, and together we can start praying for our enemies and those who persecute us. Now we have a recipe of how to make it thru this life. Time is short! Let's throw everything into this and be *transformed* by the renewal of our minds!

THOUGHT QUESTIONS

- Looking back over this week, what were some situations that occurred that caused you to be tempted to feel anger? What was your perspective of what happened?

_____

_____

_____

_____

_____

_____

_____

- How can you reframe that situation to see it from God's perspective instead of your own? How could you have changed your heart and shown more mercy in light of God's mercy on us?

  _____

  _____

  _____

  _____

  _____

- Write out Proverbs 19:11:

  _____

  _____

  _____

  _____

- How does this verse tell us to treat perceived offenses? How can you put this into practice each day? :

  _____

  _____

  _____

  _____

- Humility is being focused on God and expecting nothing from anyone. How has your stronghold(s) demonstrated a lack of humility? Think about changes in your life since you have participated in this Series. What are some indications of greater humility or dependence on God in your heart? What expectations do you have?

_____

_____

_____

_____

_____

- How does your stronghold indicate a lack of faith and trust in God as your Provider, Protector, Defender, and Giver?

_____

_____

_____

- What feeling are you looking for when you run to your stronghold?

_____

_____

_____

- How has your stronghold fulfilled that need in the long run? To the contrary, how has God provided for that feeling? In other words, describe how God can help you feel better than your indulgence. If you have not experienced this, pray for God to reveal this specifically to you.

_____

_____

_____

_____

_____

- Hebrews 4:13 says: *Nothing in all creation is hidden from God's sight. Everything is uncovered and laid bare before the eyes of him to whom we must give account.* Most of the time we do not think that God is around, but He is there with you all the time. What has often helped me stay on track in every situation is realizing that God is with me in the kitchen when I eat. He is with me when I am supervising my employees. He is with me when I talk with my husband or my children. He is with me when I am at a social event. He is with me when I am treated unfairly or wronged. I imagine Him with me in any and every temptation. When you invite God into your temptations, more than half the battle is over! I recommend that you imagine yourself looking into His pleading, loving eyes. Use the space provided to write down tempting situations where you can now start imagining God in your presence.

_____

_____

_____

_____

Luke 6:38 states: *Give, and it will be given to you. A good measure, pressed down, shaken together and running over, will be poured into your lap. For with the measure you use, it will be measured to you.* This verse explains the mysterious and ironic concept that after we give, we will get back more than we ever were trying to grab for ourselves. How can this concept help us with giving up our strongholds?

_____

_____

_____

_____

_____

_____

- What are some positive things that you could be doing for others rather than indulging yourself?

  _____

  _____

  _____

  _____

  _____

- Look again at how often your mind wanders to your desires. How does this differ from when you started? Are you finding the pull decreasing? How often is your mind wandering to or craving your stronghold?

  _____

- How is this different from when you started?

  _____

- What additional changes are you making that have led to this difference?

  _____

  _____

  _____

- Read the following passages:

  But you, brothers, are not in darkness so that this day should surprise you like a thief. You are all sons of the light and sons of the day. We do not belong to the night or to the darkness. So then, let us not be like others, who are asleep, but let us be alert and self-controlled. For those who sleep, sleep at night, and those who get drunk, get drunk at night. But since we *belong to the day, let us be self-controlled, putting on faith and love as a breastplate, and the hope of salvation as a helmet. For God did not appoint us to suffer wrath but to receive salvation through our Lord Jesus Christ. I Thessalonians 5:4–9*

It is God's will that you should be sanctified: that you should avoid sexual immorality; that each of you should learn to control his own body in a way that is holy and honorable, not in passionate lust like the heathen, who do not know God; and that in this matter no one should wrong his brother or take advantage of him. The Lord will punish men for all such sins, as we have already told you and warned you. For God did not call us to be impure, but to live a holy life. Therefore, he who rejects this instruction does not reject man but God, who gives you his Holy Spirit. Make it your ambition to lead a quiet life, to mind your own business and to work with your hands, just as we told you, so that your daily life may win the respect of outsiders and so that you will not be dependent on anybody. I Thessalonians 4:3–8, 11–12

After reading these passages, how much effort do you think we should put into the pursuit of a holy life?

_____

_____

_____

_____

_____

_____

- Remember that these battles will soon be less intense, and as time passes, you will experience only occasional temptations that do not have the intensity of your current battles. The fire will die out if you do not fan the flame. Make sure you are clearing your mental schedule for this journey, for nothing is more important than learning to love God with all of your heart, all of your mind, all of your soul, and all of your strength.

COUNTING YOUR BLESSINGS

Recognizing the countless blessings God has given you will be so important on this journey! Recount all the ways that God has blessed you, given to you, cared for you, and helped you. The more you fill in this list every day, the less magnetized you will be toward your stronghold. Spend extra time on your knees and on your face in prayer before the Father. Cry out to God and praise Him for letting you find Him and talk directly to Him. Think about it—it is so difficult to get close to famous people...yet here is the richest, most famous, most talented, and most well-known Being in the Universe, and He wants to hear from you, and He longs to have your love. Praise God for allowing you to get close to Him! Focus this week on the heavenly Father and Jesus Christ, and you will have a great week as you learn to approach each day, minute by minute, hour by hour!

COMMON STRUGGLE FOR LESSON 7

You have come a long way on this journey of letting go of your strongholds and seeking only God. One of the things you have learned along the way is the wonderful protection and fulfillment that God provides for the people who love Him…and the devastating destruction and emptiness experienced by those who hold onto worldly idols and do not put God first in their lives. A common problem that we have every week, especially in this country, is that we are exceedingly aware of the kindness of God (it is taught constantly in our churches), but we are not aware of the severity of God. Romans 11:22 states, *Consider therefore the kindness and sternness of God: sternness to those who fell, but kindness to you, provided that you continue in his kindness. Otherwise, you also will be cut off.* By this point in the Strongholds Series, you have probably noticed that God is using every emotion possible to move you to make Him the Lord of your life. He uses love and fear, happiness and sadness, and blessings and curses. It is time to acknowledge the mercy God has shown you throughout your life as you have stumbled and taken the wrong paths. Turn your face toward Heaven and do not look back!

PRAYER

Dear God, please forgive us that we do not just melt before you when we study your handiwork and your wisdom throughout the world. Please grant us patience for perseverance. Any gift we have must be developed to glorify you. Any relationship we have must be worked on to reflect more of your love and your kindness and your forgiveness. Help us to realize that this is just a normal part of the journey towards your heart. Help us to realize that we are pleasing you by seeking and following your will. Thank you for your grace and your mercy. In Jesus's name, Amen.

POSITIVE HEART AND BEHAVIOR CHANGE LIST

Write down your positive heart and behavioral changes. Some changes will be emotional or mental, some will be spiritual, and some will be related to your physical and spiritual strength. Think and write, then think and write some more! Let God open your eyes to the ways this strongholds program is affecting you and the people around you.

_____

_____

_____

_____

_____

_____

_____

_____

_____

_____

_____

_____

_____

_____

_____

_____

_____

_____

_____

_____

_____

LESSON 8

FREE TO LOVE GOD

SCRIPTURES

- [ ] Psalm 94:19
- [ ] I Peter 5:7
- [ ] II Timothy 1:7
- [ ] I John 4:18
- [ ] Hebrews 13:6
- [ ] Isaiah 41:10
- [ ] Philippians 4:6
- [ ] John 3:1-8

- [ ] II Corinthians 7
- [ ] I John 5:1-4
- [ ] II Thessalonians 2:11-12
- [ ] John 14:15-31
- [ ] Romans 12:2
- [ ] Romans 8:5-6
- [ ] I Peter 2:4-10
- [ ] Jeremiah 2:20

WEEKLY CHECKLIST

- [ ] Watch Lesson Eight Video
- [ ] Answer Lesson Eight Homework Questions
- [ ] Use your Reinforcement Resources

REINFORCEMENT RESOURCES

- [ ] *Weigh Down TV*—Watch Revolution Lesson 2, "You Are Loved"
- [ ] *Weigh Down TV*—Watch "Ambassadors for Christ"
- [ ] *Weigh Down TV*—Watch "Desert Oasis 2019—Victimization"
- [ ] *History of the Love of God*—Read Chapter 27, "Greater Love has No One"

THOUGHTS FROM THIS LESSON

Write down the revelation and make it plain on tablets so that a herald may run with it. For the revelation awaits an appointed time; it speaks of the end and will not prove false. Though it linger, wait for it; it will certainly come and will not delay. Habakkuk 2:2-3

This world is in troubled times from a lack of faith and an abundance of prophesied curses from Deuteronomy 28. We have seen dramatic increases in hate, terrorism, alcohol consumption, tobacco and drug use, family discord—all of this combined with a rise in mental health issues and world-wide economic suffering. The pain is global, because trust is disappearing, and fear is creeping into the world. When God is set aside, revenge rises into the hearts of mankind...and revenge breeds retaliation...and retaliation breeds violence. When there is a growing distance with God, humanity follows their own desires, which lead to acts of the sinful nature: sexual immorality, impurity, debauchery, idolatry, witchcraft, hatred, discord, jealousy, rage, selfishness, dissent, factions, envy, drunkenness, orgies, and the like as it says in Galatians 5:19-21. Everything starts to crumble.

But take heart! Even with all that is occurring locally and globally—all the hatred, the substance abuse, the relational problems, the financial problems—there really is *hope*! The answers are here if you know the Truth! God's Truth will free you from the fears and anxieties that come from a world led by man.

This will be a journey. To break free from the magnetic pull of the world and its man-made, self-serving answers, you must walk thru several doors. This journey does not start with a large army...it starts with *you*; it starts inside each individual's heart. Each person is so valuable, and you would not be here if God had not called you. Now is the time to fully enter into the Kingdom of God. This is not a time to take a few steps forward and then look back; it is time to give your heart to God all the way. You have been thru much warfare—and I know it has increased since you began taking this *Freedom from Strongholds* Series! You must recognize that satan has been after you so strongly because of one reason: it is because you are extremely important to God. Read that again and take it to heart: you are extremely important to God.

It all starts with the Source of all matter and life. God is Everything, and when you truly consider that concept, it inspires you to pull yourself up and focus on Him and everything He wants. This process starts inside of you. Sin is crouching at your door, but you must master it.[1] You have been waiting for something to happen that will fix everything, or for someone to say something that will make everything right, but this must come from within you—**you** must make the choice to embrace personal responsibility, because the Kingdom of God is within you.[2]

Everyone who believes that Jesus is the Christ is born of God, and everyone who loves the father loves his child as well. This is how we know that we love the children of God: by loving God and carrying out his commands. I John 5:1-2

If this is love for God, then start today, this minute. Do not wait for something else to happen. Faith means that you act first thru your obedience. Faith means you change first, and then God gives to you.

TAKE THIS TO HEART:
YOU ARE EXTREMELY IMPORTANT TO GOD!

Faith is an action. *"You have faith; I have deeds." Show me your faith without deeds, and I will show you my faith by what I do. James 2:18* James made it very clear that faith and actions cannot be separated. Jesus stated, *If anyone loves me, he will obey my teaching. My Father will love him, and we will come to him and make our home with him. John 14:23b.* Again, faith is shown thru actions: if we love Christ, we will obey him.

I cannot believe that I have been given an opportunity to live this life…and then to have the possibility of God in me? Of Christ in me? The chance to have the Holy Spirit of God inside of me? Rejoice if you have even a little softness in the stone of your heart so that you can open

---

1   *If you do what is right, will you not be accepted? But if you do not do what is right, sin is crouching at your door; it desires to have you, but you must master it. Genesis 4:7*
2   *The kingdom of God does not come with your careful observation, nor will people say, "Here it is," or "There it is," because the kingdom of God is within you. Luke 17:20a-21*

it and cry out to God, "God, I do not want a heart of stone. I want a heart of flesh. I want to start over. I want to love!" Your faith is that you have repented, you have taken action to make things right before God. *Put to death, therefore, whatever belongs to your earthly nature: sexual immorality, impurity, lust, evil desires and greed, which is idolatry. Colossians 3:5* The flesh will only make you desire more and more, eventually leading to the point where you cannot stop. But if you put these earthly desires to death, then God comes in and makes His home with you, and then you have the victory...*for everyone born of God overcomes the world. This is the victory that has overcome the world, even our faith. I John 5:4* This victory includes God's Spirit living inside of you—the Spirit of love, joy, peace, patience, kindness, goodness and faithfulness and self-control from Galatians 5. You receive joy inside of you, love inside of you, all of these amazing characteristics. That is priceless! You are letting God know you are never going to turn away from Him again. You are faithful and will

---

TO FOCUS ON CHRIST FOR THE PURPOSE OF IMITATION OF HIS RESPECT, COMPLIANCE, AND LOVE OF SERVING GOD IS A *JOY*!

---

wait on His signals. You have your heart set on God's commands, and you long to show Him that you love Him more than yourself.

You will be truly transformed thru this faith and thru your new focus. Going thru the testing, the suffering, the trials, oh yes! That is a part of it! Tested, tested, tested and retested. We discussed the Desert of Testing earlier in this Series, and you know that anything worthwhile is not going to be easy or simple. It is going to take all that you have, but that is just normal. Why do people stumble? They stumble because of their own desires. In I Peter, we learn: *As you come to him, the living Stone— rejected by men but chosen by God and precious to him—you also, like living stones, are being built into a spiritual house to be a holy priesthood, offering spiritual sacrifices acceptable to God through Jesus Christ. For in Scripture it says: "See, I lay a stone in Zion, a chosen and precious cornerstone, and the one who trusts in him will never be put to shame." Now to you who believe, this stone is precious. But to those who do not believe, "The stone the builders rejected has become the capstone," and, "A stone that causes men to stumble and a rock that makes them fall." They stumble because they disobey the message—which is also what they were destined for. I Peter 2:4-8*

There is no more time for stumbling. We have come too far and are not going to do that. I know that you can do this. You are obtaining the life-giving Spirit of Truth that sets you free so you can run and walk and be transformed and be totally born again, walking in newness of life. You are going to have a whole new life, a whole new personality, a whole new outlook. Everything changes!

An important warning to remember is that our American society is growing increasingly greedy—many believe that they truly deserve more...they deserve to reward themselves for any suffering they are going thru, they deserve to be angry with others, they deserve to indulge themselves. And of course, as we learned, this mindset only brings more pain. They have their own solution for their pain: disconnecting from the Mainframe Computer, disconnecting from God Almighty. What these hurting people do not realize is that by doing this, they are causing their suffering, not solving it. That lie of "rightful disconnection" is not good. It leads to death. We do not deserve to indulge ourselves beyond God's boundaries. We do not live to please ourselves; we live to please the Father. Every hour is God's hour, and every day is God's day. This is God's body and His time. He has such amazing plans for you! He had plans for all those evenings when you were indulging yourself. He had plans that were amazing! It is time to give God back the whole day, including His evenings and His weekends. This Connection to God is everything, and it is built upon love. *Long ago you broke off your yoke and tore off your bonds; you said, "I will not serve you!" Jeremiah 2:20* We are not going to do that any longer. We are going to get connected and stay connected thru Jesus Christ and thru fellowshipping with a true body of believers who are also connecting thru Christ.

Notice that the animals God created obey His will, just like the Angels in heaven. Yet mankind as a whole stops to consider their own selfish will far too much. People want to tear off the bonds and not be under God's authority...to their own demise. If only everyone would realize that to focus on Christ for the purpose of imitation of his respect, compliance, and love of serving God is a *joy*! Christ's entire life is to be copied because it is one unbroken continuum of selflessness to the service and for the glory of God, lived out in love and for the eternal welfare of all the brothers and sisters—for all mankind. Jesus is the author of this Connection, living and dying showing us how to turn away from our evil desires and connect to the Source of all life permanently. Jesus was all in. *The world must learn that I love the Father and that I do exactly what my father has commanded me. John 14:31*

Always keep in mind, especially now that you have been thru warfare, you are extremely important—God loves you!—and that reverses the lie satan whispers that you are not valuable. *You are loved.* You have been loved on. You have been given life. You are destined to live forever and ever in this love. And God is love.

The truth is, God has been shortchanged. You loved the world more than Him. And that has been the problem...you have been loving the wrong thing. So what was in your heart was every practice of man and his evil desires. It is time to rally! *Do not love the world or anything in the world. If anyone loves the world, the love of the Father is not in him. For everything in the world—the cravings of sinful man, the lust of his eyes and the boasting of what he has and does—comes not from the Father but from the world. The world and its desires pass away, but the man who does the will of God lives forever. I John 2:15-17*

It is time! What better way than to learn from history so that it will not be repeated. It is time for overdue glory to The One True God, The LORD God Almighty, and His Son, Jesus Christ who is at the Father's right hand. May God's Kingdom come and His will be done on Earth as it is in Heaven. It is time to give the throne back to the rightful King and **go all in** for His Kingdom!

THOUGHT QUESTIONS

- Reread Deuteronomy 28 in light of this lesson. The signs of a lack of faith and the increasing curses line up with what we have been seeing in the world in recent years. What are some of the changes and situations you have noticed in the world—and in your own household—that are also indicators of the curses in that passage?

_____

_____

_____

_____

_____

_____

- On the other hand, over the course of *Freedom From Strongholds,* what are some of the blessings you have personally experienced as you put into practice the lessons you have learned from this Series? List all the blessings you can think of, no matter how small or large! Grab another journal to continue adding to this list.

_____

_____

_____

_____

_____

_____

- How have you controlled your evenings in the past for your own interests and indulgences? Make a plan today to give God back His nights and weekends. What are some practical things you can do when you are tempted during the evening hours or weekend "free time"? (For example, pray to God for His plans, read His Word, watch the video lessons or do the workbook lessons, reach out to others to encourage them, serve your family or neighbors in some way, take care of household needs, etc.)

_____

_____

_____

_____

_____

_____

• Now record the results after putting the above into practice. How did you feel the next morning after spending the prior evening seeking God's plans instead of giving in to selfish desires? How was God's way more fruitful? (For example, falling asleep peacefully with no guilt about wasting the evening, getting more done around the house which made your family happy, etc.)

_____

_____

_____

• Write out James 2:18 below:

_____

_____

_____

• What do your deeds over this past day or week show God and others about your heart?

_____

_____

_____

- Review the list of strongholds in the Bible passages below and the ones on page 13-14 in this workbook. As you review, think about the progress you have made and some areas in which you need to go further in laying down.

  ☐ Romans 1:26-32   ☐ Mark 7:22-23
  ☐ Galatians 5:19-21   ☐ II Timothy 3:1-5
  ☐ Ephesians 4:29-5:5   ☐ Colossians 3:5-10

- After reading thru these passages, what are some areas in your life where you know God is still trying to get your attention? What are the areas you can improve on? Are there other strongholds you need to work on laying down next?

  _____

  _____

  _____

  _____

  _____

  _____

- Over the course of this Series, we have learned even more how God is truly *everything*. What does it mean to you to acknowledge God? What does that look like day-to-day in your own life?

  _____

  _____

  _____

  _____

  _____

  _____

- Read Numbers 14:32–34. How long did God tell the Israelites they would remain in the desert because of their unfaithfulness?

  _____

- Think about the journey of God's children thru the desert after the Exodus. If you have not been struggling in your hot desert of suffering for over 40 years, know that you have not suffered any longer than the Israelites, and know that it is perfectly fine to go over and over the heart material that is in this course. Heart material is very different from intellectual material, and perhaps it needs to be applied every day for the rest of your life to help you on this eternal, all-important quest. Go back thru your workbook lessons, re-watch the video lessons, re-take the Series as many times as you need to fully turn your heart, soul, mind, and strength to the Almighty God!

COUNTING YOUR BLESSINGS

Recognizing the countless blessings God has given you will be so important on this journey! Recount all the ways that God has blessed you, given to you, cared for you, and helped you. The more you fill in this list every day, the less magnetized you will be toward your stronghold. Spend extra time on your knees and on your face in prayer before the Father. Cry out to God and praise Him for letting you find Him and talk directly to Him. Think about it—it is so difficult to get close to famous people...yet here is the richest, most famous, most talented, and most well-known Being in the Universe, and He wants to hear from you, and He longs to have your love. Praise God for allowing you to get close to Him! Focus this week on the heavenly Father and Jesus Christ, and you will have a great week as you learn to approach each day, minute by minute, hour by hour!

_____

_____

_____

_____

_____

_____

_____

_____

_____

_____

COMMON STRUGGLE FOR LESSON 8

After making your way thru this Strongholds Series, you may be wondering: Is it possible that some strongholds are simply harder to quit than others? Generally, all strongholds are alike because they are all, basically, a heart problem and a focus problem. The cure for all strongholds is the same, as you have seen in this Series, and all can be broken free from, as you have witnessed thru the many testimonies and hopefully experienced to some degree yourself. The length of time someone has been in a stronghold does have some influence on the strength of that stronghold's pull because it has become so routine; the stronghold has become a years-long habit. However, the repentant heart can break thru—sometimes within one day, never to look back—even if the person has spent 50 or 60 or more years in the stronghold. I have seen it happen! However, the most damaging thing you can do to a relationship with God is waver back and forth repeatedly from the idol to God. This is dangerous because of the damage it does to the confidence on either side of the relationship. The person can lose self-confidence, and, more importantly, God can lose confidence in the person, and He can become very jealous.

The privilege of choice is incredible. Those of us currently living in the United States live in a free country; we have not experienced the level of burdensome enslavement or oppressive governments that some people have. Therefore, we often do not see the urgency to make the right choice and seal it with wholehearted devotion. We think we will always have another chance, another option. But know that it will get harder and harder to build and keep this relationship with God if you play around with it. What husband tolerates his wife going from one affair to another, coming home only to go right back out into adultery? Why do we think God responds any differently? I will tell you why— it is because we do not truly know Him or His personality. The Bible tell us clearly: *...my people are destroyed from lack of knowledge. Hosea 4:6* This is referring to a lack of knowledge of God's personality. We do not truly realize what makes Him angry or happy, and even though it is written right there in His Word, we have not cared enough to find out. It is time for this casual mentality to end. We cannot play around with the convicting information that God has given us. Look for His peaceful path and walk in it. And once you put your hand to the plow, do not look back. You will be so richly blessed.

PRAYER

Dear Lord, help us realize the strategic importance of only having One Love. Help us to realize the importance of focusing on this lifelong journey as our number one priority. God, you are love, and love will come back to us if we will devote our heart, soul, mind, and strength into adoring you and your Kingdom. That is your promise to us in your Word. Thank you for being such a great God. Lead us not into temptation, and deliver us from all evil, for yours is the power and Kingdom and the glory forever. Amen.

APPENDIX

ADDITIONAL RESOURCES

All available at www.WeighDown.com

Weigh Down Ministries is the non-profit publishing house for, and is sponsored by, Remnant Fellowship Churches. It has been producing resources for over 30 years which have proven to help participants overcome overeating, alcoholism, gambling, drugs, sexual sins, materialism, and other strongholds, fully supporting all people seeking to glorify God and promote His Kingdom. If you need help or know someone who needs help, please refer to this list of resources.

Remnant Fellowship Services

Visit a worship service in Brentwood, Tennessee. Hear powerful instruction, uplifting worship music, and testimonies from like-minded believers. Visit www. RemnantFellowship.org to learn more!

Weigh Down on Tour & Remnant Regional Gatherings

Check our online calendar on RemnantFellowship.org and WeighDown.com to see if Weigh Down is coming to a city near you.

Gwen Shamblin Lara Library

For a Complete List go to www.GwenShamblinBooks.com

Weigh Down Works!

This 30th Anniversary edition expands on the basic principles of The Weigh Down Diet and includes more tips and many encouraging success stories.

The Weigh Down Diet

National Best Seller. Original book by Gwen Shamblin Lara, written in 1992. Practical advice to help you on the path from physical hunger to spiritual fulfillment.

Rise Above

A follow-up book to *The Weigh Down Diet*. Look inward into your own heart and learn to transfer your devotion to the food over to a wholehearted devotion to God Almighty.

The Legend To The Treasure

This book contains powerful spiritual lessons on how to lay down the last bit of self and praise of man, coupled with practical, true statistics of what life is like without God.

Dig deeper into your life—find out if you are pursuing the True Treasure, and find an inexpressible joy that comes from a relationship with God alone.

History Of The One True God Volume I: The Origin Of Good And Evil

Beautiful and clear account of Genesis Chapters One through Eight and how these events affect us to this very day. Hear the history of lucifer's fall from Heaven, the creation of the world, Adam and Eve, Cain and Abel, and Noah from the perspective of the great love the Creator has always had for mankind and the great appreciation that is due Him in return. Audio book available exclusively on Store.WeighDown.com.

History Of The Love Of God Volume II: A Love More Ancient Than Time

An inspired writing that starts with a history of God's love for man and mankind's appropriate love back to the Father, then explains how this True Love can overflow into love for those around you (even the unlovable)! A must have for every family.

History of the One True God Volume III: God-Fearing Families

This book will give you the practical steps you need to make the dream of a loving, united, God-centered family a reality for you and your loved ones.

Weigh Down Classes

Classes are available on WeighDownTV, and have an accompanying workbook, audio lessons, and reinforcement lessons. If you need help selecting a class, call us at 800-844-5208 or email us at info@weighdown.com

Weigh Down Basics

Six-week beginning class which teaches the foundational principles of WeighDown. Learn how to eat like a Thin Eater between hunger and fullness, end greed eating and emotional eating, and end dieting by learning how to change your focus off of food. The result is permanent freedom from overweight!

Exodus Out Of Egypt: The Change Series

Eight-week weight loss class that goes beyond the basic foundational principles of WeighDown Basics and The Last Exodus. Including practical tips, hints, and advice on weight loss and dealing with "problem" foods or tempting situations during the day.

Weigh Down Chats with Gwen

A 9-episode series that teaches how to make permanent changes while gaining a deeper understanding of the purpose of your life, your goals and what we are all working towards.

Breakthrough

Eight-week advanced weight loss class for those who have already been through our other classes but have plateaued in their weight. This class will emphasize personal accountability and responsibility and will help you truly let go of all control and learn to let God lead ALL the way.

Greed Exposure

This 9-week online class will help you control overspending, manage your budget and eliminate your debt.

History Of The One True God

Six-week class of the great love shown by God for all created beings and the appreciation due Him in return. A moving study which will strengthen your relationship with God more than ever before.

The Legend To The Treasure

Sixteen-week advanced class for the last bit of weight or self-focus—based on nautical symbolism that helps the participant steer his ship in the right direction toward a deeper relationship with God. A deeper look into the world we live in, providing insight to what we truly treasure and adore.

Weigh Down Advanced or "Remnant Basics"

Ten-week class—discover the root of any remaining pull toward your strongholds and take your relationship with God to the next level. This opens your eyes to the big picture of how rebellion affects God and His Church.

Feeding Children Physically & Spiritually

A practical guide for children, parents, and parents-to-be for healthy childhood development.

For a complete list of marriage, parenting and strongholds resources, go to Store.WeighDown.com

WEBSITES & FREE RESOURCES

Weigh Down TV

Become a member now! This service provides unlimited streaming to Weigh Down classes and class materials with an extensive library of videos and audios on all subject matters including marriage, parenting, depression and more. Sign up today. Visit WeighDown.TV or download the app on your mobile device or TV to join!

WeighDown.com

Visit our website for the most up-to-date information on coming attractions, media events, frequently asked questions, free weight loss lectures, special events, and many testimonies! Sign up to receive weekly emails.

GwenShamblinLara.com

Learn more about author, Gwen Lara, her family, and the founding of Weigh Down and Remnant Fellowship.

RemnantFellowship.org

More information on Remnant Fellowship Church, which sponsors Weigh Down Ministries. You will find many inspiring testimonies, videos on what we believe, and access to our live worship services. E-mail questions to info@remnantfellowship.org.

Twitter

Follow "GwenShamblinLara" and "WeighDown" for uplifting encouragement.

Facebook

Follow Weigh Down, Gwen Shamblin Lara and Remnant Fellowship on Facebook and join the Weigh Down Ministries Facebook Group—the 24/7 newsfeed is filled with testimonies, encouragement, sharing, and answers from the office. This group is a great way to stay connected and be encouraged anytime you need fellowship and friends who will point you up to God!

WeighDownRadio.com

Weigh Down Web Radio (WDWB) provides free 24/7 online encouragement. Hear testimonies, music, and Godly instruction by Gwen. This is a wonderful resource to have playing in the background while working around the house or cooking in the kitchen! Go to weighdownradio.com.

YouTube

Watch inspiring videos on the GwenShamblinLara, RemnantFellowship and WeighDownWorkshop YouTube Channels. Be sure to visit the LifeWithGwenandJoe channel to learn more about Gwen and Joe!

GwenShamblinBooks.com

A complete library of Gwen's books.

For more information, please call us toll free at 1-800-844-5208 or visit WeighDown.com.

YOU ARE NOT A FAILURE

You are not a failure! You have simply been applying the wrong remedies to try to be free from your strongholds. For three decades, Gwen Shamblin Lara had the opportunity to work personally with tens of thousands of people who applied the principles laid out in her program and as a result, found freedom from a wide variety of unhealthy habits and strongholds. Gwen's teaching began in the field of weight loss, but God's Truth can be applied to all areas of life, and His Truth sets you free. For permanent change to be successful, God needs to be involved; after all, He is the true Creator of

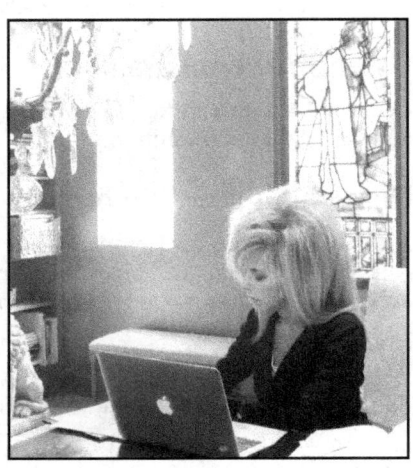

the concept of behavior modification. We were made to master this.[1] Thru countless classes, seminars, and writings, this teaching has reached millions, and the statistics are unprecedented. These long-term results are not to be found at any medical clinic or weight loss facility in the world. Any program can possibly produce a few

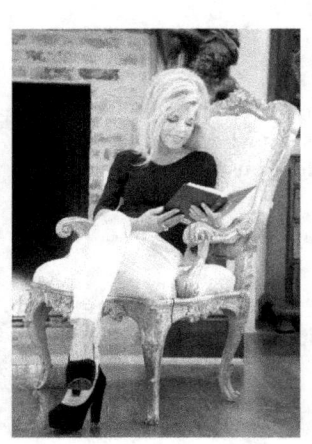

testimonies of people who happened to lose weight or stopped smoking or had a healed marriage, but no other program has produced thousands of testimonies who have maintained that success for three, five, ten, or even twenty years! Yes, something is very different here, and it should give you much hope! The testimonies you meet on our websites and in our materials are everyday people just like yourself—they had tried everything possible to stop overspending, end eating disorders, stop overdrinking or smoking, end illicit drug use, regain endless hours spent on video gaming or social media, and exchange a life of anger for a life of peace... only to return to their past behaviors after the latest attempt was unsuccessful. But then they tried just one more time thru Weigh Down or Strongholds...and they learned the secret of how to turn to God for help on His terms. It truly makes all the difference, as you are about to see for yourself!

---

1   *If you do what is right, will you not be accepted? But if you do not do what is right, sin is crouching at your door; it desires to have you, but you must master it. Genesis 4:7*

About Gwen

Gwen Shamblin Lara, M.S., R.D, was a registered dietician with a Master's degree in food and nutrition. She was a member of the American Dietetic Association with five years of experience working in health departments and then another five years of experience as an instructor of foods and nutrition at the University of Memphis.

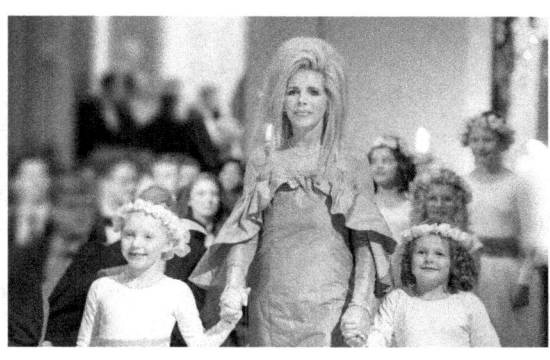

A very spiritual person with a strong faith in God, Gwen felt led to found The Weigh Down Workshop in 1986 in order to teach the Godly principles you will learn in this program to those who were desperately seeking to lose weight permanently. Initially offered thru audiotapes and small classes taught by Gwen in a retail setting, this teaching began yielding unprecedented results. Participants were not only losing excess weight while eating regular foods, but they were using the same Bible-based principles to turn away from other strongholds, such as smoking, marital discord, financial debt, or alcohol abuse.

By 1992, the Weigh Down program was packaged for seminar use, churches began to sign up, and the media began to pay attention. The growth was explosive. By the late 1990s, Weigh Down was internationally known in most Protestant, Catholic, and Evangelical churches around the world. Gwen Shamblin Lara and The Weigh Down Workshop were featured on such shows as 20/20, Larry King Live, and The View, as well as in such magazines as Good Housekeeping and Woman's Day. In

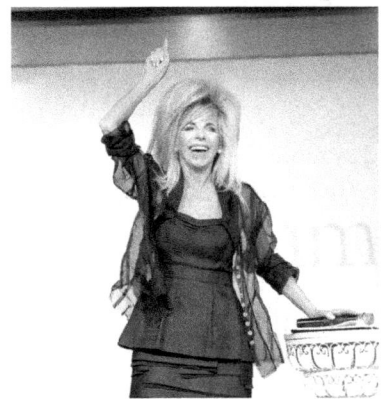

1997, Gwen's first book, The Weigh Down Diet was published by Doubleday, Inc. The book quickly sold over one million copies as people discovered the secrets to losing weight quickly and permanently while discovering a new relationship with God. Gwen's teaching was called "revolutionary" by the media, where she was coined as the "Pioneer of Faith-Based Weight Loss."

Over the last 30 years, Weigh Down has freed thousands from excess weight without dieting or over-exercising. Countless people

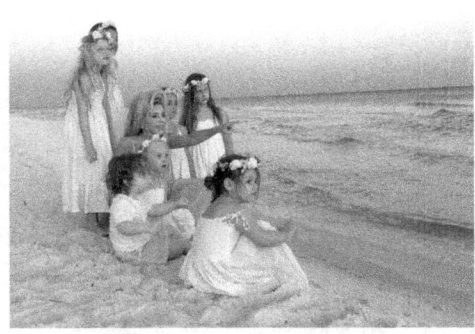

have been set free not only from the pain of overeating and eating disorders, but also from other addictions and harmful habits. After Gwen's success, many faith-based programs have copied her fundamental teachings, but neither Gwen nor Weigh Down's success has ever been duplicated.

In 1999, Gwen, along with several other families who were seeking to re-estab-lish the foundation of the early Christian church, founded Remnant Fellowship Church. This small gathering has continued to grow over the past two decades and is currently a flourishing Christian church providing services across the world for all ages.

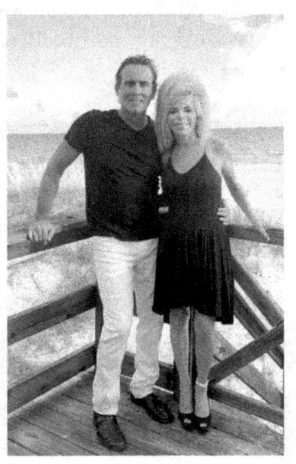

Gwen enjoyed a fun and God-focused life with her husband, Joe Lara, which can be seen in their video series "Life with Gwen and Joe," available on YouTube. Gwen raised two children and enjoyed eight grandchildren. Gwen's son, Michael, has four children with Elle Shamblin, and Gwen's daughter, Elizabeth, has four children with her husband Brandon Hannah. They have always been supportive of Gwen's teachings, and their contributions have been invaluable.

Gwen, her husband Joe, her son-in-law, Brandon, and four very close friends were tragically lost in a plane crash on May 29, 2021. Gwen's legacy will continue for generations as she has a place in the hearts of millions of people around the world thru her work with Weigh Down Ministries and Remnant Fellowship Church.

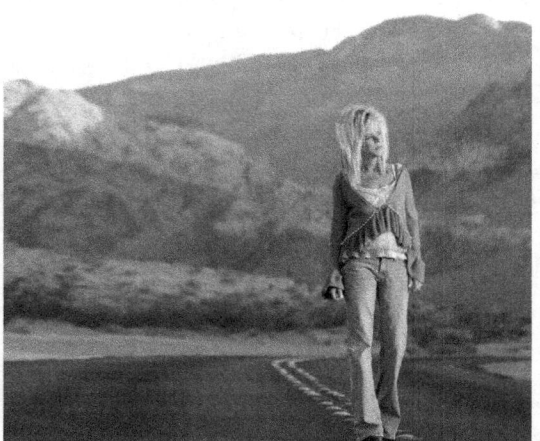

For more about Gwen, please go to GwenShamblinLara.com

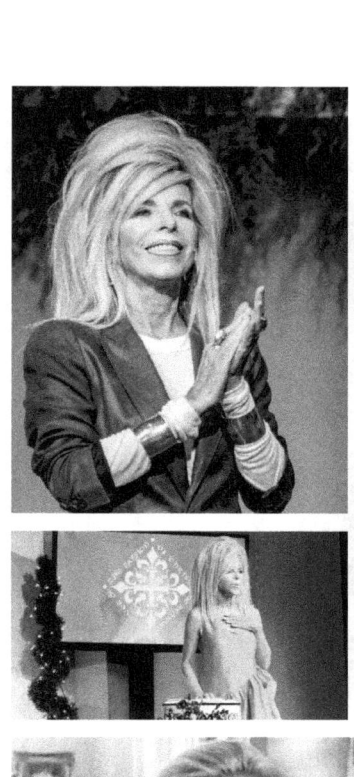

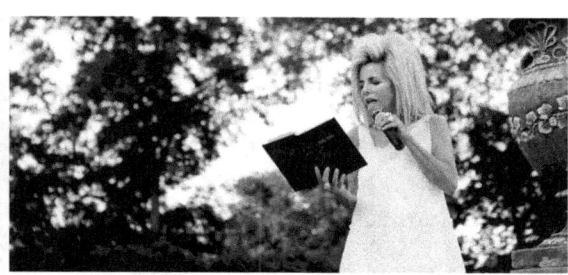

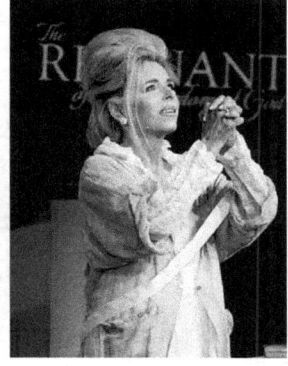

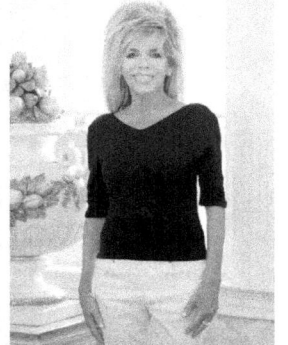

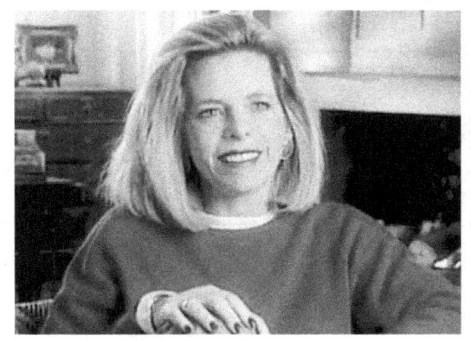

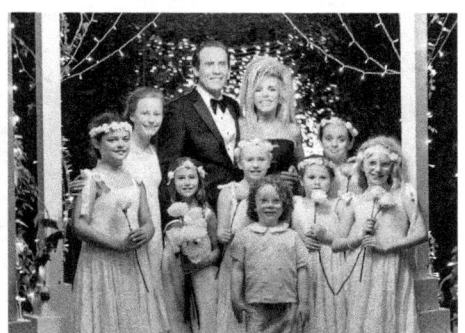

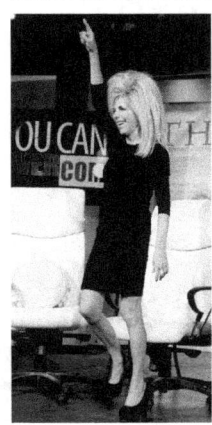

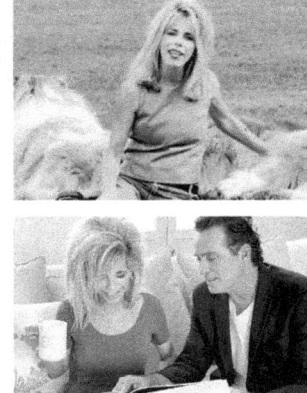

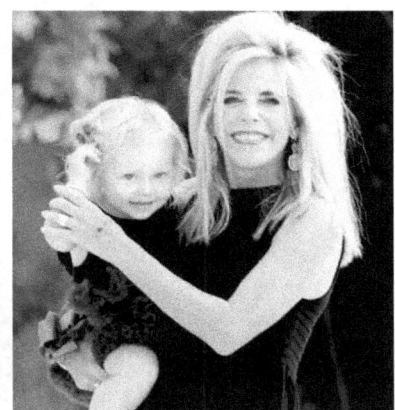

CPSIA information can be obtained
at www.ICGtesting.com
Printed in the USA
LVHW051302200423
744589LV00001B/2